# The Practitioner as Teacher

## THIRD EDITION

*Edited by Sue Hinchliff*

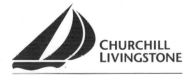

CHURCHILL
LIVINGSTONE

EDINBURGH  LONDON  NEW YORK  OXFORD  PHILADELPHIA  ST LOUIS  SYDNEY  TORONTO  2004

CHURCHILL LIVINGSTONE
An imprint of Elsevier Limited

First edition 1992 by Scutari Press
Reprinted by Baillière Tindall and copyright transferred 1996
Second edition 1999
Third edition 2004

ISBN 0 443 07286 8

**British Library Cataloguing in Publication Data**
A catalogue record for this book is available from the British Library

**Library of Congress Cataloging in Publication Data**
A catalog record for this book is available from the Library of Congress

**Note**
Medical knowledge is constantly changing. Standard safety precautions
must be followed, but as new research and clinical experience broaden our
knowledge, changes in treatment and drug therapy may become necessary
or appropriate. Readers are advised to check the most current product
information provided by the manufacturer of each drug to be administered
to verify the recommended dose, the method and duration of
administration, and contraindications. It is the responsibility of the
practitioner, relying on experience and knowledge of the patient, to
determine dosages and the best treatment for each individual patient.
Neither the publisher nor the editor assumes any liability for any injury
and/or damage to persons or property arising from this publication.
*The Publisher*

 your source for books,
journals and multimedia
in the health sciences
**www.elsevierhealth.com**

The
Publisher's
policy is to use
**paper manufactured
from sustainable forests**

Printed in China

# Contents

learning; The adult learner; Androgogy and pedagogy; Superficial versus deep learning; The importance of individual differences; Motivation; The value of reflective practice to the teaching and learning process; The importance of journal, log or diary writing to learning; How to write a journal; Recording your journal; Linking theory with practice: the role of the practitioner; Teaching strategies; Building the framework: why we need a teaching strategy; Teaching a skill; Preparing your teaching; Communication skills; The use of humour in teaching; The what of teaching; The importance of evidence-based practice; The why of teaching; The when of teaching; The where of teaching; The how of teaching; Providing a structure for teaching; Aims and objectives; Identifying what to teach; Identifying your aim for the session; Formal and informal teaching; Deciding what to teach; Different approaches to teaching; Creating a good environment for teaching; Teaching methods; Handouts; Delivering a lecture; Discussion and tutorial groups; Audiovisual aids

Introduction; Learning objectives; Overview of competence; NHS KSF core dimensions; Specific dimensions; Development review; Linking the development review with the NHS KSF; Accreditation; Standard/competency setting; Dissemination of the standards/competencies; Comparison of the evidence; Review and evaluation

Introduction; Learning objectives; Defining terms; Evaluation as a process; Why do we need to evaluate?; When is the best time to evaluate?; Where is the most appropriate place to evaluate?; What is it we need to evaluate?; Who are we going to evaluate?; How to evaluate teaching; Self-evaluation; Gaining feedback; How to evaluate learning; Peer evaluation; Evaluating the effectiveness of your teaching; Evaluating and assessing competence; The value of learning in and from practice; What is competence and why do we need to measure it?; Assessing competence pre- and post-registration; Mentor responsibilities; Mentorship preparation; Assessing competence: the NVQ/SVQ framework; QCA as a regulatory body; Awarding bodies; Approved assessment centres; Different supporting roles; NVQ/SVQ structure; Choice of units; Teaching and assessing – getting started; Route planning

# List of contributors

**Anne Eaton**  BSc RN RM RCNT RNT Cert Ed D32–35
Programme Director, Skills for Health

**Sue Hinchliff**  MSc BA RN RNT
Head of Accreditation, Royal College of Nursing of the United Kingdom, London, UK

**Sue Howard**  MA RN DNCert RHV DNT
Acting Assistant Director (Education), Royal College of Nursing of the United Kingdom, London, UK

**Sally Thomson**  MA(Ed) BEd(Hons) RN RMN RNT
Director of Nursing and Clinical Effectiveness, Oxleas NHS Trust, Kent, UK

# Dedications

**Anne Eaton**   *to Mum – for supporting me and believing in me*

**Sue Hinchliff**   *to Philip, Katy, Charlie and Alfie – for your love*

**Sue Howard**   *to my grandson James – a lifetime of learning and love*

**Sally Thomson**   *to Bill and Gilly – my greatest teachers*

# Preface

In the 13 years since the first edition of this text there has been much change. Contextually, the government has changed, which has brought changes to the NHS and the health care agenda in the UK. Devolution has taken place, which has meant that health care is no longer – if it ever was – delivered in a homogenous way throughout the UK. The regulatory body has changed, as has the initial preparation for practice. Education has changed generally, and nurse education in particular with a much greater emphasis on competence, fitness for practice and lifelong learning.

This has meant that this book has had to change – considerably. The third edition bears little resemblance to the editions that went before. It is common, with continuing editions of a book that has earned its position in the market-place, simply to tweak existing chapters for a new edition. This might mean a few additions to further reading; some fresh references and adding in allusions to changes in legislation or new trends. For this text now though, that would not be enough, so we have started anew, but with the same contributors who have themselves moved on to different positions in the health care world.

There are five new chapters with an altered focus, but with learning and teaching as paramount threads. The focus is on the practitioner and his or her learning journey. We hope that you will enjoy travelling that journey, with this text to signpost the way.

Sue Hinchliff
London, 2003

# 1 Creating a learning environment

*Sally Thomson*

## INTRODUCTION

The potential of learning in practice settings is extraordinary. Learning is the most powerful medium for change, and when that change affects the quality of patient care it is compelling. To ignore learning opportunities for those who care for patients and clients means that practice and individuals will not move forward. Regardless of how we learn, the process increases self-esteem and contributes to morale. Mix this with the idea that you yourself are both teacher and learner, and you have a powerful cocktail.

The focus of this chapter is to persuade you to consider and address your own learning needs in order to meet the needs of others in your practice setting, be they patients, carers, doctors, student nurses – in fact, any member of the caring team.

( Learning and teaching opportunities present themselves in many guises, from lengthy formal courses with an academic credit rating, to a single day spent with an expert practitioner or nurse consultant, observing practice, solving problems, talking through a clinical situation, or an hour's clinical supervision. These are all powerful tools for exploring the dynamics of practice.)

---

**LEARNING OBJECTIVES**

After reading this chapter you should be able to:

◆ Identify your pathway towards lifelong learning

◆ Explain the knowledge-base from which you teach in the clinical setting

◆ Discuss the use of evidence-based practice and intuitive practice

◆ Identify the positive factors in your clinical area and those you need to develop to foster a positive learning environment

◆ Consider how you might bring about a change in culture that encourages a learning climate.

---

## TEACHING NURSING

**ACTIVITY 1.1**  Before you start this section, you may wish to note down some key words that reflect what nursing in your specialism means to you. Do this before reading the next section.

Regardless of whether you are teaching a colleague, or are a pre- or post-registration nursing student, what you are actually transmitting is an advancement of a nurse's understanding of practice. In 2003, after extensive consultation, the Royal College of Nursing (RCN 2003) developed a core definition of nursing with six key characteristics, in which it is claimed lies the uniqueness of nursing. The definition takes account of the diversity of nursing, admits that some parts can be shared by other professions, but asserts that nursing uniquely combines these six attributes. Nursing is:

> 'The use of clinical judgement in the provision of care to enable people to improve, maintain, or recover health, to cope with health problems, and to achieve the best possible quality of life, whatever their disease or disability, until death' (RCN 2003).

The RCN defines the key characteristics as:

1. **A particular purpose**: to promote health, healing, growth and development, and to prevent disease, injury and disability. To minimise distress and suffering and to help people understand and deal with their disease or disability, treatment and outcomes. If death is inevitable, then to maintain the best possible quality of life.

2. **A particular mode of intervention**: to enable people to achieve maximum independence. Nursing practice is an 'intellectual, physical, emotional and moral process' which includes the assessment of nursing needs, nursing interventions and personal care. It involves information, advice, advocacy and 'physical and emotional support'. Nursing practice also includes management, teaching, policy and knowledge development.

3. **A particular domain**: to focus upon people throughout their lifespan and context, looking at the responses to (and experiences along) the continuum of health to illness. This will often combine physiological, psychological, social, cultural and spiritual elements.

4. **A particular focus**: the whole person and the human response.

5. **A particular value base**: nursing is founded on ethical values, 'respecting the dignity, autonomy and uniqueness of human beings, the privileged nurse–patient relationship, and the acceptance of personal accountability for decisions and actions'.

6. **A commitment to partnership**: with carers, patients and relatives all interchanging the role of leadership with team membership. However, the nurse is at all times personally and professionally accountable for decisions and actions.

The significance of defining nursing as above is reflected in the way that nurses work in modern health care systems, and the way that practitioners are prepared. This links directly with how you prepare practitioners for the different levels of practice in your clinical setting.

Now return to your notes about nursing from Activity 1.1, and try to link your ideas to the six characteristics described above. Explore the above characteristics for your area of clinical expertise. For instance, if you work in child health, the domain of nursing is clear. Children's nurses have values in terms of family care. The responses to situations would depend upon the patient's level of psychological maturity. With your personal application of this definition of nursing, you can begin to consider what it is you might be teaching in your specialism and what you may need to learn for your own development. Finally, complete this section by considering who your students will be. The modern approach to teaching and learning is to share the experience throughout the caring professions. Many workforce confederations commission joint programmes of learning. Some universities run a multidisciplinary foundation course, with the professional groupings forming after the core learning has been achieved. It may be worth exploring what happens in your area, as the possibilities for joint learning and teaching are immense.

Your answer must reflect the rich mix of students that you have – those who wish to develop skills but who are less experienced than yourself in your specialism; traditional students on pre- and post-registration nursing courses; health care assistants studying for National Vocational Qualifications (NVQs), or carrying out care under your supervision; members of the multidisciplinary team who, in this climate of shared learning, recognise that there is much to learn from each other. This is the beginning of a very complex teaching and learning matrix.

## THE CHANGING EMPHASIS ON LEARNING

There has always been an emphasis on nurses teaching in the practice setting, but today there is a strong focus on the need to develop a culture of learning and teaching in the workplace.

The term 'lifelong learning' came into popularity with the Dearing Report on Higher Education (National Committee of Inquiry into Higher Education 1997). The main principle of this report is that if we each take responsibility for our own learning and development, we will create a learning society. The report's underpinning philosophy is that people from all walks of life should continue with training and education, in order to keep abreast of the rapid changes taking place in our lives and in the world.

Nurses are aware of the constant development and updating needed to maintain their knowledge and nursing expertise, as the rate of change and development in health care and health policy is so rapid.

**ACTIVITY 1.2**

Stop for a moment, and note down some of the issues that you believe all the nurses in your team need to learn about in order to keep abreast of change. Try to think of your own learning needs as you do this.

You may have noted a whole range of issues relating to the definition of nursing, and also to changing treatments and technology, research, generating evidence for practice, or updating your computer skills.

An additional emphasis on learning from 1995 was the requirement for nurses to maintain knowledge and skills in order to remain on the register. The Post-Registration Education and Practice Report (UKCC 1997) – known as PREP – significantly changed the attitude of registered nurses towards their own learning. A large part of your role as teacher may be directed towards creating and contributing to an environment that promotes such learning.

**ACTIVITY 1.3**

This is a good point for you to explore your curriculum vitae, to ensure it is up-to-date, and to look again at your portfolio. As you develop skills of teaching in the clinical setting, you will be able to broaden and deepen your portfolio. You may wish to set some objectives that will focus on your teaching skills.

The Department of Health (DoH) in England produced a document entitled *Working Together – Learning Together. A Framework for Lifelong Learning* (DoH 2001) relating to NHS modernisation. This document sets out what staff can expect from employers, focusing in particular on ensuring that the NHS has a workforce with the right number of staff, with the right skills in the right place at the right time. This clearly describes the context for teaching and learning across the health care team. The report defines the effectiveness of learning organisations, stating that learning is the key to improving working lives. The document is full of ideas for good practice, and recommends that the Trust Board should monitor the learning and development strategies linking them to clinical governance.

**ACTIVITY 1.4**

What learning and development strategies are in place for your clinical area that link into the Trust's strategic plan and objectives? If you have not seen it, get a copy of the plan from the Trust Board minutes. These are open papers, accessible from your Chief Executive's office. With the nursing team, explore how your area can contribute towards delivering the objectives of the strategy.

For example, who do you need to consult with? What will your strategy embrace? Break it down into steps.

Hopefully, you will have included the multidisciplinary team and teaching staff who are your partners in creating a learning organisation. This will give you a context in which you can focus upon your own teaching skills.

Among the many recommendations of the DoH report is the need for all staff to have an individual professional development plan (PDP). This can be achieved only as part of the annual staff development review (SDR).

**ACTIVITY 1.5**

When did you last have your SDR? (see also Chapter 4). When did you set the objectives and milestones, note your achievements, or adjust your strategy to meet your plan?

Plot the timeframes for the SDRs of the team in your clinical area. With your colleagues, discuss how a joint PDP can be drawn up for the team so that their training and education needs are clearly set out alongside a targeted improvement in performance.

The above exercise is the very essence of creating a learning environment.

*Working Together – Learning Together* (DoH 2001) discusses how professionals must continually update and extend their knowledge and skills. By mapping all those required for your clinical area, you will start to explore some of the knowledge-base required to meet training needs. The report differentiates between continuing professional development (CPD), which refers to updating of existing skills, and post-registration education, which broadens and enhances skills. The employer has a responsibility to ensure that the workforce is clinically effective, and practitioners have a commitment to lifelong learning. Underpinning the NHS Lifelong Learning Strategy is the development of a skills escalator that involves everybody in learning, from catering staff to consultants.

Lifelong learning may include opportunities for formal courses that are assessed and carry credit at a given academic level. For example, you may be reading this book as part of your studies at academic levels two or three. Equally, it embraces those informal moments when you pursue your learning for yourself, or to solve a problem at work. However, learning is an active process and will not happen unless you order, categorise and evaluate your thoughts. The joy of learning in the practice setting is that the learning can be applied directly to care, which helps your student further to categorise and process their existing knowledge. The benefit of linking theory with practice is that understanding facts – for example the physiology of the blood and the effects of anaemia on a person's functioning – comes to life when an anaemic patient describes the symptoms and experiences of the illness to a nurse, particularly if the supervising nurse then takes time to explore the pathology reports, compare them to normal values, and so on.

Lifelong learning helps to ensure that you remain flexible and open to change; in fact, it may cause you to initiate practice developments.

Finally, developing knowledge is powerful, both personally and in terms of growing confidence and professionalism, as knowledge offers an unshakeable platform for our work. Edwards (1997) begins his challenging read on this issue by quoting Foucault:

> Knowing if one can think differently than one thinks, and perceive differently than one sees, is absolutely necessary if one is to go on looking and reflecting at all. (Foucault 1987, p. 8; cited by Edwards 1997.)

Lifelong learning, then, provides the philosophy that should underpin both your personal development plan as a practitioner who continues to develop professionally, and also underpins the role that all clinicians have in transmitting their practice to others.

This may be a good point to reflect upon the development of your own portfolio. A portfolio encompasses all the experiences you have had to date.

These may be influenced by the sort of person you are, why you chose nursing as a career, and significant experiences that you have had – both in your personal life and in nursing – that have affected the way you care. A portfolio might contain contracts, photographs, leaving cards, records of achievements, performance review, role descriptions and so on. A profile is a more focused document, in which you draw from the broad portfolio aspects of yourself that you wish to portray for a particular purpose. The time when this is often used is in the 'statement in support of application' at the end of a job application, when you get a chance to map yourself against the characteristics of the role description or person specification.

| ACTIVITY 1.6 | Take out your portfolio and extract the learning experiences you have had in the past 3 years. You may wish to put these under different headings. For example, courses with an academic credit rating, starting with your pre-registration course; short courses or workshops that you have completed as part of your professional role; then, perhaps to fulfil your PREP requirements, the learning you have gained from reflection on, and making sense of, experience; and finally, a section for self-generated learning. If you have plans for the future, either formal study or knowledge and experience that you intend to acquire, it is worth logging this in your portfolio at this point. |
| --- | --- |

A portfolio is something that you return to in order to develop over a period of time as your experience grows (see also Chapter 2). This exercise will clearly demonstrate the nature of lifelong learning and the effort that needs to go into it. To compare your map with that of a peer may help you to identify gaps, either for yourself or for your colleague, and may lead to an identified learning need which, in turn, will meet client needs.

This is an important exercise, not only in terms of understanding what lifelong learning means, but also as a crucial part of your development plan. You are likely to use it as a tool for agreeing learning needs during your performance review, or as part of a job application, or for reviewing the skill-mix of the nurses in your area of practice. If you find a tool that helps with your development and also promotes the generation of ideas and discussion of issues in your clinical team, you are beginning to develop a template for making your own clinical area part of the wider learning organisation.

From this initial exploration of lifelong learning, and as you progress through this book, you will realise that learning is about change. You should now return to your portfolio of learning experiences and ask yourself what changed as a result of the learning. You will notice that some learning developed client care; some was about you; and some about learning for learning's sake. You may also have developed new communication skills, a change in self-confidence, new practical procedures, or an assertive approach.

In order to achieve this learning plan for your clinical area, you will need to think about how to coordinate, develop and sustain such a strategy, including the resources and support you will need. You must also identify the learning needs of pre- and post-registration student nurses. What results is likely to be quite a complex and detailed plan, where the responsibility for teaching and learning rests with everyone in the health care team.

The National Audit Office (NAO 2001) discussed how the quality of practice placements affected what and how nursing students learn. The NAO strongly encouraged partnerships between the higher education institutions and the clinicians who apply learning in practice. The report suggests that such close working could only benefit the student, and reduce the high level of attrition that universities experience in their nursing courses.

---

**ACTIVITY 1.7**   Reflect on the contact you have with your local university. Could you develop your role and network with educators in order to improve the quality of teaching? What might you gain from this?

Your answer to the above probably shows a rich mix of shared responsibilities. There have been many imaginative and successful measures to foster partnership and enrich the learning environment, and to emphasise that the responsibility for the student is shared between the university and the Trust. If your thoughts do not reflect this, now is the time to think through and talk to the team about your joint role in forging these links.

---

In the aftermath of the inquiry into the Bristol Royal Infirmary (Kennedy 2001), when safe care became a crucial issue, the competence of health care professionals in clinical practice came under close scrutiny. A strong recommendation was made in the report for shared learning, particularly between undergraduate medical and nursing students. Lifelong learning and CPD were major themes of the report, with practitioners needing to demonstrate their levels of competence. Clinical supervision can provide the medium for assuring safe care, with an emphasis on the development of expert practice.

## TEACHING PRACTICE INTELLIGENCE

There is an interesting conundrum about what learning you as a teacher will facilitate in your clinical area. The smart answer to this is that you will teach about your practice. But where does this knowledge come from? Now the answer gets more interesting, because it focuses on what students need to know to be able to practise in their own way as nurses.

# TEACHING USING THE PRINCIPLES OF PERCEPTION

Your aim is to transmit the way you see nursing into students' minds, so that they can understand and evaluate practice from their own perspective. There are several perceptual principles you can use to help students arrange information usefully and meaningfully in their minds and promote understanding.

Perceptual theories (Atkinson et al. 2000) tell us that how we process thoughts and understanding affects learning, particularly how we store information in memory. The trick in storage, of course, is to be able to retrieve things as and when we need them. It is useless to store your saucepans in the loft if you are going to use them every day. Similarly, what is the point of keeping old table lamps in the kitchen cupboard if you rarely need them?

Whatever it is you wish the student to learn, the student will do her own learning depending on the way in which she arranges in her mind the information you have given her. For instance, when learning we may screen some things out as irrelevant, or not comprehensible, and therefore not put them into the right 'storage box' in our minds. Checking understanding, asking questions and linking knowledge directly to your patients' experiences will help the student classify information and underpin understanding, that is, put the information into the right storage boxes.

The Gestalt school of psychology (Atkinson et al. 2000) describes perception in relation to pattern formation. This principle can help you to help others to structure their thoughts. The first principle we use when looking at patterns is similarity. In order to create a pattern, the same shapes, sizes and colours are used, so that similar elements are grouped together. In teaching, you can use this principle by beginning with what the student knows. For example, a woman asks for an explanation of her brother's pleurisy and the symptoms he is experiencing. You ascertain that she has little knowledge of body function. You might begin by describing the pleura as a petticoat, the layers gliding upon each other smoothly as the lungs move with breathing. The petticoat develops static electricity, so the smooth movement of the layers is disturbed. You would then move on to explain that the layers of the pleura are sticking together as a result of inflammation, and that this prevents free movement, which in turn causes pain. Analogies have a useful place in enhancing perceptual processes. I am sure you can think of many that were used when you were learning physiology. I have never forgotten how one tutor explained the function of the peritoneum. She stood with a straight face, arms outstretched, fists clenched, a drawsheet over her head, patiently explaining that her arms were the fallopian tubes, her fists the ovaries, her body the uterus, and the drawsheet was the peritoneum. I would not, however, recommend this in the middle of a gynaecology ward, unless you are desperate to make everyone laugh! However, if you can make learning fun, people are much more likely to remember.

Secondly, when looking at patterns we search for proximity. This is when similar objects are grouped closely together and enhance accurate perception. In clinical units, patients are grouped in this way; surgery is broken down into specialisms; mental health is broken down into the needs of the patients, with units for adolescents, forensic care and so on. This means that when you enter a clinical environment you anticipate the sort of care issues you will face. In teaching, it is possible to create proximity by demonstrating contrasting and similar properties. Suppose that you are teaching a student the principles of wound management: you may begin with an aseptic technique on a small simple wound. Next, you could perform a dressing incorporating a corrugated drain, and then you would move on to one with a vacuum on a closed drainage system. At the end, you could sit down with your student and explore the principles of care involved for the three patients, beginning with the basic principles that apply to all three and then exploring the differences.

There is continuity in a pattern when similar parts stand out, so that the basic building blocks of the pattern are evident. Continuity can be achieved with your student by moving sequentially through a topic in a logical manner. You may be supporting a student in a mental health unit specialising in affective disorders. The student has to care for a range of patients, and you may begin by exploring a normal mood with its ups and downs, perhaps caring for a patient who is recovering from depression, assessing her mood against your jointly worked out meaning of 'normal'. You may then move on to work with a client who is severely depressed, so that the student can see a continuum of mood, from happy to severely depressed. You may then go on to explore elation, and apply this to patients in your care. Continuity does not happen if, for example, you jump from mood to the Mental Health Act, to disorders of perception, the effects and side-effects of tranquillisers, and then to depression. Continuity implies an orderly progression.

The fourth principle is closure, which focuses on the fact that closed or partially closed patterns are easier to perceive than unclosed ones. This is the principle behind 'join the dots' in children's comics. By summarising a clinical session with a student, you help them to join the dots by applying theory in practice. A summary allows the integration of material discussed in the session into a perceptual pattern, tying all the threads together to give greater meaning.

**ACTIVITY 1.8**   Now consider a subject you frequently teach when caring for patients. How can you use the principles of similarity, continuity, proximity and closure to enhance this topic? Plan a short session, deliver it, and then carefully evaluate your students' learning. How could you improve on this the next time?

# LEARNING TO USE THE RIGHT KNOWLEDGE

Students need information, that is, cognitive knowledge. Most of this is taught as part of the formal process during the academic parts of the course, and assessed in this way. However, it is essential for a student to absorb how knowledge can be applied to a patient that she is caring for.

---

**ACTIVITY 1.9**

Choose a patient in your care, and begin to write a list consisting of:

- The knowledge a student needs to begin to understand the nature of the patient's problem. This may be physiology, anatomy, psychology, sociology – or a blend of all these.
- What understanding the student needs of the patient's condition. Again, this may involve an explanation of a surgical intervention, or pharmacology to understand the effects of medication, or details of the patient's lifestyle, and so on.
- The therapeutic intervention you and the student are about to undertake – what information does the student need about this?

---

As you explore this with the student, you are both using cognitive knowledge to develop understanding and also psychologically arranging things to promote the principles of perception. Keep this instance firmly in your mind as you work through the rest of this section.

Remember, even though a student has covered the theory through formal teaching and learning methods, rehearsal of information will strengthen the perceptual state of readiness or mindset that you are trying to create.

Cognitive learning requires us actively to process information. This happens when existing knowledge mixes with previously learned material to create new knowledge, so creating an assimilation of facts.

Now return to the list you began to compile above. You are going to care for a patient, so how will you elicit the student's knowledge and understanding?

# TEACHING FROM EVIDENCE-BASED PRACTICE

You will be aware of the move to underpin all aspects of care with a rationale based on evidence. This requires skill in assessing evidence, analysis, decision-making and reflection. The first issue of an evidence-based journal (Editorial 1997) describes evidence-based nursing as giving quantitative or qualitative meaning to the cause, course, diagnosis, treatment and economics of health problems managed by nurses, including quality assurance and CPD.

It is one facet of theory underpinning practice, by integrating research into practice.

Knowledge exists in many different forms, and emerges from a variety of (often opposing) research disciplines. Therefore, both the planning and the teaching of best practice for patients rest on your clinical expertise, patient preferences and research evidence.

This may be a good point to stop and note how many interventions you make based on research evidence, adding this to the list you are compiling for Activity 1.9.

Start small, and find one area where you could expand your portfolio and validate an area of your practice. This will undoubtedly mean visiting the Internet or your nursing library.

# LEARNING AND DEVELOPING SKILLS

This aspect of learning is concerned with practical competence – giving an injection, bathing a baby, using equipment. Practical skills are to do with movement, so although developing relationships is an essential skill it is not a psychomotor skill.

In every clinical area there are psychomotor skills that are either specific to that area, or general to many placements.

You could devise a matrix that illustrates both the skills a student needs to achieve the competencies in your area, and other skills that can go on being developed during a placement in your specialism.

Returning to your list in Activity 1.9, think about what skills you are going to use during the episode of patient care. Establish whether the student is competent or unpractised in those skills. Then you can plan observation, rehearsal or supervised practice when with the patient, and can develop the student's perceptual set by cueing her to observe specific aspects.

Vicarious learning occurs when you do not realise what you have learned until you need to demonstrate the behaviour. Think of how easily a little girl is able to apply her mother's lipstick to understand this approach! Learning by watching the behaviour of others is powerful. Observe the outcomes that the behaviour produces for others, and assimilate this into memory (Atkinson et al. 2000). Complex patterns of behaviour can be acquired in this way, and even emotional responses can be developed by watching others. An angry parent will unconsciously teach a child to cope using aggression, and an assertive parent offers a completely different repertoire of behaviours.

Now go back to your list (which by now must be getting quite complex). Can you identify behaviours you are going to model? By now, your list should have the essential knowledge the student needs in order to make sense of, and perceive accurately, the session on care, the skills needed, and an expectation of the social behaviours you will model. It will be useful, after digesting the next section, to look back and see if your predictions were correct and to analyse what you learned.

# LEARNING AND TEACHING FROM EXPERIENCE

This is what teaching in the practice setting is all about, and it is useful to acknowledge that the distinction between personal and social learning is blurred. Experiential learning reflects the student's own perception and understanding of a situation. It can develop moral, professional and personal understanding.

Benner (1984), in her classic work, identifies how students pass through five levels of proficiency, ranging from novice to expert (see also Chapter 2). Benner's work clearly indicates the sensitivity of the theory–practice gap, and clearly points to the need for teaching in the practice setting. It may also give you some clues on how to approach your teaching. For example, the novice moves to a ward after a period in college. While in this placement, the novice is actively learning rules and the principles of basic skills. The skills are inflexible – novice students are unable to contextualise them – that is, they are unable to make small adjustments to skills to apply them in practice.

The advanced beginner demonstrates a marginally acceptable performance. Benner suggests that a mentor might have helped her to cope with sufficient situations to enable the student to apply the rules.

The competent practitioner will have been in role for 2 years or more; she is consciously aware of her actions, has the feeling of mastery, but lacks the speed and flexibility of the proficient nurse. Benner advocates that a mentor can help this nurse by helping to plan and coordinate complex care situations.

The proficient nurse has a deep understanding of the situation, in that she experiences it as similar to past experiences stored in memory, and in this way a plan develops unconsciously.

Finally, Benner's expert has an intuitive grasp of each situation and is able to select and analyse a problem without consideration of the alternative aspects. An example is a ward manager who, seemingly intuitively, advises the night staff to watch a patient closely and predicts a sudden change in condition, which then materialises.

You may easily be able to identify colleagues in these categories across the multidisciplinary team. This will help you consider their learning needs, and also how they can support you with yours.

One of the most significant and relevant ways of maximising the benefits of a clinical placement is to teach from the experience your student is having.

There are two ways of using this – both have a structure. One tends to be more teacher driven, using an experiential learning cycle; the other is a tool that all practitioners should use: a reflective process. Both lend themselves to the processes of mentorship and supervision, and are excellent and effective for understanding and processing experience.

Miles (1987) describes the process of an experiential learning cycle. The first stage is personal experience; for example, you may arrange for a student to observe an aspect of care. Before the care episode, you sit down with the student to explain the nature of the care and particular things to look out for. Then, you share perceptions from the experience. What did you observe? What did you feel? It would be useful here to turn the description into key words, as these will aid retention of the event.

Next, you must move on to make sense of the experience: the student needs to understand what it all means in order both to inform and illuminate future care. Concepts, generalisations and principles can be abstracted by exploring to what extent this patient's experience is typical of other patients, perhaps using the key words to identify similarities and differences. Finally, you could encourage the student to think of other situations, and to plan the care for a different client.

Experiential learning is equally valid for a first injection, the birth of a baby, breaking bad news or handling an emotional outburst.

Reflective cycles share similar properties. Boud et al. (1985) describe how to use a learning experience using a reflective model. The model has three phases: the experience, the reflective processes, and the outcomes. Practitioners can use this model independently, or in tandem with a facilitator.

First, an experience is identified that is worth exploring. The events are replayed, usually in a written format, but this can be verbal or visual. The practitioner in the second stage has to focus upon the feelings associated with the experience, including the identification of behaviours and ideas. Then the nurse processes the emotions to sort and make sense of both the negative aspects for future care, and the positive elements of the experience. This re-evaluation of positive and negative issues cements the learning that has taken place.

Finally, in the third stage, by reflecting on the previous dynamics the practitioner is able to create new understandings and applications.

**ACTIVITY 1.10**

Consider how you can use the two models. Go back to Activity 1.9, where you identified what knowledge the student needed in your area, and add 10 more aspects that could be enabled using an experiential learning cycle or reflective process.

Next, with a colleague, identify a situation that you both agree is worthy of reflection, use the model, work through it individually, and then compare notes.

In the above exercise together you will have discovered some interesting revelations and differences. You may each identify different features that are positive and negative. Much of this is due to individual differences in values. You may even see a situation quite differently, one seeing the negative as positive, and vice versa. You may wonder if you both witnessed the same event. In the discussion on perception, we explored how to understand a situation. This is crucial to learning. So, understanding how two people see a situation from each other's perception can also be critical to effective learning.

Valuable personal experiences can be created in groups, or in one-to-one settings. Although learning through reflection is a powerful medium, like all methods it has its pitfalls.

Schon (1987), a classic writer in this area, contends that personalising and reflecting on experiences enables the student to transfer professional knowledge to 'real world practice', enabling them to progress through Benner's five stages. Schon discusses at length the notion of professional artistry, describing it as a form of intelligence, a kind of knowing, although different from professional knowledge. Artistry is evident when competent practice is demonstrated in conflicting situations.

Schon calls this 'knowing in action'. He contends that 'reflection in action' will develop this professional artistry, building a bridge between theory and practice. Reflection, then, is something that you can facilitate in others and develop yourself. It is worth reading Bolt's (1991) work on *Becoming Reflective* (see Recommended Reading).

## TRANSMITTING YOUR INTUITIVE KNOWLEDGE

All experienced nurses can recall an incident where they used intuitive judgement, or observed another nurse doing it. Think of the clinical nurse who convinces a psychiatrist to test the thyroxine levels of a depressed patient, and has what appeared to be a hunch proved correct when the patient is found to have hypothyroidism. Or take the midwife who senses a postpartum haemorrhage is about to happen, or a health visitor who knows that a child is at risk.

An important part of experienced-based practice that Benner (1984) felt was the distinguishing feature of the expert nurse, is intuition. Benner held that this evolves from a blend of knowledge, skill and practice, and therefore encompasses the broadest of knowledge bases. There is, as you will have read earlier, a drive for evidence-based practice which conflicts with theories of intuition and the benefit of the latter in nursing practice.

Intuition has been described as a 'gut feeling' (White 1996), and so it seems an intangible concept that is difficult to investigate.

Definitions clearly link intuition with experience. Dreyfus and Dreyfus (1986) describe the understanding that effortlessly occurs upon seeing similarities with previous experiences – based not on guesswork, but on sound knowledge. Intuition in practice, therefore, involves the recognition of previously experienced patterns (perception) and the detection of subtle clinical changes. It is recall partly from past experience that emerges as a form of reasoning, developed as we practise. The significance of helping students to perceive clinical situations accurately, and to store this perception in memory, is strong.

If we use intuition, we are able to take shortcuts in complex situations. Cioffi (1997) links this rapid reasoning to the subtle processing of probability, making subjective judgements that enable practitioners to develop shortcuts. These reduce a complex situation to a more simple operation of judgement. Cioffi suggests that intuitive knowing involves drawing on experience, experiencing feelings of knowing, sensing subtle qualitative changes, and linking perceptions from the past with expectations of the future. This perceptual awareness enables the experienced nurse rapidly to separate out relevant from irrelevant information, and to understand the situation as a whole (pattern perception) rather than as a series of tasks. This removes the need for deliberate analysis of a range of information. She suggests that, when using intuition, practitioners draw on both theoretical and practical encounters. The danger, of course, is that a misdiagnosis is made. You only have to think of the question and answer technique that doctors use to understand that it can be fraught with difficulty. Particular symptoms may close off a perceptual pattern too quickly, and vital clues may be missed which would lead to a different diagnosis.

White (1996) links personal intuition with both research and practice, suggesting that this combination of knowing offers the best for those we care for. We often see intuition used in emergency situations, where rapid information processing and rapid response are both significant to the patient's recovery.

Intuition involves a range of responses, knowledge and the use of Gestalt theories of perception, so that patterns form the basis for thinking and the ability to predict, which permits us to suspect a change before it happens.

**ACTIVITY 1.11**

Reflect upon a clinical situation where you used intuition. Note down what happened. What resources do you need to draw upon in order to teach this 'knowing' to a colleague?

This is a difficult task, but if we can teach from our intuitive self we can transmit expert practice to others.

You may have drawn on a knowledge-base, but you have also thought about approaches to different styles of learning and have been able to unpack some of the contextual events around this experience.

# LEARNING USING ALL THE DOMAINS THROUGH SUPERVISION AND MENTORSHIP

Helping others learn depends on the principles of effective communication. The teaching style that practitioners tend to adopt is that of a professional conversation. The nature of teaching in practice revolves around finding out what the student knows, transmitting what you know to build on that, and to apply that knowledge directly to the care you are giving. The relationship that you build with your student is crucial to the learning dynamic. The communication styles you adopt, and your ability to ask the right sort of questions at the right time, will all influence what the student learns. This includes:

- Listening and responding effectively

- Helping the student to identify feelings and personal knowledge

- Sharing yourself and your intuitive practice as well as thoughts and feelings

- Being sensitive to the student's needs

- Being aware of your personal strengths and weaknesses and their effects upon others.

The skills could form the basis of the supervision that you receive, and a large element of your reflective writing if you are a diary keeper.

These professional relationships can be a part of supervision and mentorship. Although the principles of these helping relationships are similar, there are differences – the most obvious is that, in most Trusts, mentors are linked with unregistered students and supervision usually explores the practice of the registered nurse.

**ACTIVITY 1.12**

The subtle differences are worth exploring. Follow the guidance on mentoring and supervision used in your place of work, as well as your experience of each way of working. If you do not have a copy of the guidance in your workplace, the higher education institution will have one. Either the Registry or the link lecturer will be able to provide it. Compare and contrast the two approaches, mentoring and supervision. If you find it difficult, ask a colleague to share the work with you. Alternatively, this could become a project for those whom you facilitate. This links directly to the teaching and learning matrix you have been forming throughout this chapter.

You will see that differences lie in the nature of the relationships formed, in the process, in the ways of overseeing, in the formality of the relationship, in the style of evaluation and in timeframes. You will have also discovered that there are many similarities between the two processes, and that many registered nurses get confused about the specifics of each way of working. A team seminar may be useful to clarify this for others, and to raise issues that need addressing in your area.

Brereton (1995) found that the most effective bridge over the theory–practice gap was the mentor's insight into and understanding of the mentoring role.

By now, you will have realised that in all teaching sessions you are likely to teach from behaviourism, knowledge and intuition, using the rewards that form part of social learning theory, for example as you smile, nod and value a student's contribution.

## CREATING A CLINICAL LEARNING ENVIRONMENT

The social context of work and a person's ability to learn are directly related. Hart and Rotem (1995) conducted a study to identify the attributes of effective learning environments in clinical settings. It would not be surprising to note that some clinical environments are more effective than others, and organisational and social factors play a key part in this. The authors identified six factors that contribute to a positive learning environment:

1. **Autonomy and recognition:** the extent to which staff are valued, acknowledged and encouraged to take responsibility for their own practice

2. **Job satisfaction:** the extent to which nurses enjoy their work and intend to pursue a career in nursing

3. **Role clarity:** the extent to which staff understand and accept their role and responsibilities

4. **Quality of supervision:** the extent to which supervision and staff interaction facilitates or impedes improved practice

5. **Peer support:** the extent to which staff are friendly, caring and supportive of one another

6. **Opportunities for learning:** the extent to which learning opportunities are restricted or available.

There are some clear messages for all practitioners from this research. Each of us in practice is responsible for the contribution we make to the clinical culture, and it only takes one or two shining lights to achieve a change in culture and create a learning organisation. Handy (1993) describes how innovation and change are natural outcomes of reflection in and on practice, which all practitioners are encouraged to undertake within a learning organisation. Handy describes the organisation as having the 'E' factor: excitement, enthusiasm, effervescence and energy.

Organisations learn only through individuals who learn. Individual learning does not guarantee organisational learning. But without it no organisational learning occurs (Handy 1993).

A learning organisation, then, allows the staff to learn and grow both personally and professionally.

**ACTIVITY 1.13**

- Consider whether your unit is a learning organisation in miniature.
- Does it have a belief or philosophy about nursing? Either at unit level or for the Trust?
- Does it have stated aims and objectives, and a clear direction for care?
- Does everyone understand the way forward for care?
- Do you have any learning facilities? Noticeboard, flip chart, books, a room to use, access to professional journals?
- Does someone in the team have the role of training coordinator? Does that person link to the higher education institution?
- Is there a staff development system that is apparent at clinical level? Do you have your performance reviewed, are training needs identified, and are these linked into the team's needs?
- Are training needs met and evaluated?
- Are staff encouraged to discuss and exchange ideas?
- Is leadership visible?
- Are patients encouraged to offer their views, and contribute ideas on the provision of care?

If you cannot answer with a positive yes to the above questions, you have some work to do.

Begin by examining the culture of your clinical setting. Malim and Birch (1998) describe this as a system of meanings and cultures shared by an identifiable group. To assess a learning environment accurately, it is important to consider the influence of the culture that has developed and the reasons for the direction it has taken. The culture is crucial to the way we are socialised into work, and is something you should think about when orientating new staff. Within a culture, subcultures may develop that also have attitudes, values, laws and codes of conduct.

Socialisation is the process by which people become part of the culture; it is the process by which we learn how different groups work (Malim and

Birch 1998). It is a lifelong process that helps us deal with new experiences. This is an important concept for a learning organisation, where you can effectively socialise colleagues into the values that underpin the organisation and its way of being. Each person can then affect the behaviour of others by the way they interact and transmit messages about values.

The power of conformity and compliance is strong, and it is useful to understand this when working to develop a new culture. Conformity occurs when members of a group behave similarly to other members of that group. Consider the enormous pressure on new student nurses to adapt. Once new entrants into a care setting have assessed the prevailing values, they are able to relax and join the group, developing a sense of belonging. If a dominant value is difficult to pinpoint, people become anxious. The unconscious need to conform is so strong that it can even affect how and what we eat (Norman et al. 2001). The power of effective leadership here is obvious.

Compliance is a more complex concept. It occurs when members of a group behave in the same way as others, even if they feel uncomfortable doing so. Consider the scapegoating of individuals that can occur as a result. For instance, suppose an influential leader is negative about the skills of a doctor. Because of this, the rest of the team may respond in a negative manner. Reverse the situation: consider how popularity is promoted, and carries along with it a tide of contagious goodwill. The danger or strength of compliance (in a healthy environment) is that eventually a person may come to adopt the values that underpin the compliant behaviour and conform! The need to conform and comply is a powerful tool to utilise when trying to build your learning organisation. Orientation programmes, briefings, debriefings, giving feedback on performance – these are all examples of the efforts made to bring about conformity and compliance perceived as desirable.

This may be a good time to refer to a basic social psychology book, and to refresh your memory on the dynamics of groups. Malim and Birch (see Recommended Reading) are enjoyable to read.

Attitudes are the next aspect that you will have to consider when working to create your learning organisation. Attitudes are described as having three parts: thinking, feeling and acting. The thinking part of an attitude is supported by beliefs, such as 'smokers are self-destructive'. The feeling part of an attitude refers to the emotion that is associated with that behaviour: for example, you may be repulsed by cigarette smoke. The acting element is the behaviour that goes with it: opening a window, sighing if someone lights a cigarette, moving away from the smoker. The three aspects of an attitude tend to be consistent, and are learned aspects of our behaviour that make us behave in certain ways.

However, supposing a very attractive person lights up a cigarette on a date: you may hate the smell but stay close, thinking you will change this person if the relationship lasts! Actually, it is you who will change. When you shake the foundations of one aspect of an attitude, you will strive for consistency with the other two elements so that you are comfortable with yourself and your values.

From this point of view, changing attitudes can be achieved by reasoned argument and persuasion. Even so, they are difficult to alter.

If you use the power of conformity and compliance, you may have some success. If you can change emotions in an attitude, you have a strong chance of success as feelings act so powerfully on our thinking and behaviour. Frequent repeats of a message to change attitudes are effective, but it can take time for you to weaken the hold of one of the three elements.

## CHANGING INTO A LEARNING ENVIRONMENT

It is impossible to think about creating a learning culture without considering the dynamics of change and its processes.

First, it is essential that everyone in the team can work out what changes need to be made, and how they will recognise that these changes have happened. A lot of energy needs to go into this phase, so that everyone has a chance to feel ownership of the project. If people are anxious, or feel they do not have the right skills, these factors may be powerful forces in the resistance movement. You need to assess carefully what you can do to change such an attitude. Communication and feedback at this stage are essential.

Once you are on target with your programme, there is often a phase when things you had not anticipated happen. Perhaps the night staff have not been briefed, or someone has returned from sick leave unaware of what is happening. If there are several problems, people can become anxious and feel that they lack the skills to meet the objectives. Uncertainty requires confidence, and a conviction that the new way is better. Clinical supervision is a crucial tool here. After the wave of anxiety comes a period of maintenance. You need to keep the momentum going to manage the transition and refine the process, so that you achieve the learning environment that you believe will make a difference. Gradually, the new way will be accepted as the group norm. You may still, of course, have resistors, but compliance and conformity are strong dynamics to work with. Even so, disgruntled or anxious staff need to be managed carefully and valued during their period of resistance. As well as the resistors, you will have staff members with high enthusiasm who want the change to happen yesterday! While harnessing this enthusiasm, it is essential that these motives are managed – mixing personalities in working groups is one way to even the pressure and enable skilful team building.

It is essential to respect all viewpoints, even those of people who sit on the fence. A lot can be done to build on the energy of emotions. It is obvious that this change needs to be discussed at team meetings, and to explain that your manager is supportive of the objectives. If not, you have some attitude change to achieve. Also, it helps to hold clinics away from the team, where it is safe for people to pop in and voice their views and have their opinions heard and respected.

## CONCLUSIONS

Learning domains rarely stands alone: cognitive learning often involves emotions; reflective practice may revolve around a situation where a skill is being practised and a crucial patient interaction achieved. Facilitating learning in your environment involves social psychology, sociology, the art and science of teaching, a strong understanding of nursing, and the courage to have a go.

## REFERENCES

Atkinson RL, Atkinson RC, Smith EE, Bem DJ, Nolen-Hoeksema P. Introduction to psychology. Texas: Harcourt Brace, 2000

Benner P. From novice to expert. Menlo Park, CA: Addison Wesley, 1984

Boud D, Keogh R, Walker D. Reflection: turning experience into learning. London: Kogan Page, 1985

Brereton ML. Communication in nursing: the theory–practice relationship. Journal of Advanced Nursing 1995; 21: 3114–3324

Cioffi J. Heuristics: servants to intuition in clinical decision-making. Journal of Advanced Nursing 1997; 26: 203–208

Department of Health. Working together – learning together: a framework for lifelong learning. London: DoH, 2001

Dreyfus HL, Dreyfus SE. Mind over machine: the power of human intuitive expertise in the era of the computer. New York: Free Press, 1986

Editorial. Evidence-based Nursing 1997; 1: 7–8

Edwards R. Changing places? Flexibility, lifelong learning and a learning society. London: Routledge, 1997

Handy C. Inside organisations: 21 ideas for managers. London: BBC Books, 1993

Hart G, Rotem A. The clinical learning environment: nurses' perceptions of professional development in clinical settings. Nurse Education Today 1995; 15: 3–10

Kennedy I. The report of the public inquiry in children's heart surgery at the Bristol Royal Infirmary 1984–1995: Learning from Bristol. London: HMSO, 2001

Malim T, Birch A. Introductory psychology. London: Macmillan, 1998

Miles R. Experiential learning in the curriculum. In: Allan P, Jolley M, eds. The curriculum in nursing education. London: Croom Helm, 1987

National Audit Office. Educating and training the future health professional workforce for England. London: National Audit Office, 2001

National Committee of Inquiry into Higher Education. Higher education in the learning society (the Dearing Report). London: HMSO, 1997

Norman A, Parrish A, Birchenall P. Not so happy at work. Nurse Education Today 2001; 21: 83–85

Royal College of Nursing. Defining nursing. London: Royal College of Nursing, 2003 www.rcn.org.uk

Schon DA. Educating the reflective practitioner. San Francisco: Jossey Bass, 1987
United Kingdom Central Council for Nursing, Midwifery and Health Visiting. PREP and you. London: UKCC, 1997

White J. Midwifery: the balance of intuition and research. New Zealand College of Midwives Journal 1996; October

# RECOMMENDED READING

Bolt E. Becoming reflective. London: Distance Learning Centre, South Bank University, 1991
*An imaginative distance learning pack that enables you to explore what it is to reflect in and on your practice*

Malim T, Birch A. Introductory psychology. London: Macmillan, 1998
*An enjoyable refresher into the importance of social psychology*

# 2

# The learning and teaching journey

*Sue Hinchliff, Sue Howard, Anne Eaton*

## INTRODUCTION

This chapter describes the learning journey for both yourself and the students you are charged with teaching and supporting in practice. It explores some of the key elements of education that underpin your role as a teacher and then goes on to offer some practical ways for how you can capture evidence of the learning that takes place in practice. This is set within a framework of professional development and lifelong learning.

---

**LEARNING OBJECTIVES**

After reading this chapter you should be able to:

◆ Identify and discuss the issues influencing nurse recruitment in the UK

◆ Have an awareness of the NVQ/SVQ system and how it operates

◆ Outline the relationship between nursing and higher education

◆ Identify and discuss the outcomes and competencies of pre-registration education

◆ Have an understanding of the relationship between professional development and lifelong learning

◆ Recognise an expert practitioner and the stages on the journey to becoming one

◆ Have an awareness of the attributes of expertise

◆ Understand what is meant by lifelong learning

◆ Identify ways of capturing evidence of learning in practice.

---

# PART 1: THE LEARNING AND TEACHING JOURNEY TO LICENSED PRACTITIONER

## RECRUITMENT AND RETENTION

Most health care professions are having difficulty in recruiting to pre-registration programmes, and in retaining those students who do commence study. This scenario is made worse in nursing when we realise that after the end of their 3-year pre-registration programme some successful candidates do not register with the Nursing and Midwifery Council (NMC) and therefore do not practise as registered nurses. The government recognises that the biggest issue challenging the health service today is a lack of human resources, bearing in mind that it takes 3 years to train a nurse (DoH 2000a).

It has been recognised that approximately 1 million people work for and within the NHS, and the government spends around £2 million a year on supporting education and training for clinical staff, a large proportion of whom are nurses (DoH 2000b). On a typical day in the NHS there are:

- 300 000 nurses
- 150 000 health care assistants (HCAs)
- 22 000 midwives
- 10 000 health visitors
- 105 000 practice staff, including nurses, in GP surgeries (DoH 2000a).

These figures do not include nursing students, owing to their supernumerary status.

The figures demonstrate the size and complexity of education and training across nursing, and the sheer volume of support needed to recruit and retain such a large and potentially mobile workforce. However, the NHS Plan states that 'NHS staff are a precious resource. They are what makes the NHS tick' (DoH 2000a, p. 55).

---

**ACTIVITY 2.1**

Consider a 'normal' day in your care setting: list the numbers of staff who are on duty, and list those staff according to professional background. What are your findings?

I think you may have found that the majority of staff on duty are registered nurses, with HCAs following a close second.

---

According to the NHS Plan (DoH 2000a, p. 25) the public wanted to see more staff and new ways of working, which paradoxically included 'bringing back Matron'; the staff wanted to see more staff, alongside more training for staff.

---

**ACTIVITY 2.2**

Are there any 'modern matrons' employed in your area, perhaps in your Trust or Primary Care Trust? Find out what their roles are. Ask them the extent to which they have made a positive impact on overall care delivery.

---

Ultimately, with an achievement date set for 2004, the government intends to increase the number of nurses by 20 000. These numbers will be achieved by encouraging nurses to return to the profession, with a promise of increased flexibility, family-friendly working practices and better conditions. Many NHS employers and their colleagues in the independent sector have attempted to attract nurses back to work, with varying degrees of success.

## OVERSEAS RECRUITMENT

There is also recruitment into the UK of nurses trained and educated in other countries, again with varying degrees of success. Some see this measure as short termism, in that a large number of these registered nurses will move elsewhere, often back to their home country, and perpetuate the recruitment and retention problems in the UK.

Nevertheless, internationally recruited nurses will need the skills and experience of registered nurses to support them in their new roles and in potentially very different cultures and environments from those they have left. Registration with the NMC is not automatic for nurses who undertook their nursing programmes outside the European Union (EU): such nurses will be assessed on an individual basis and most will need to undertake periods of supervised practice and assessment before they can access the NMC register. Such staff may be employed as HCAs or 'non-registered staff nurses' in order to progress through their programmes.

According to the erstwhile United Kingdom Central Council (UKCC 2001), 'the number of applications for registration with the UKCC from overseas has trebled in the last 2 years'. The bottom line is that anyone wanting to work as a registered nurse in the UK must, in law, first register with the NMC (ex UKCC). The reason for this is, ultimately, protection of the public. All applicants must complete the relevant documentation available from the NMC, and upon receipt of this NMC staff will assess whether or not the education and training and experience of the individual applicant equips him or her to carry out the duties of a registered nurse in the UK. To facilitate this process the individual will have to provide details of pre-registration education and training, both theoretical and clinical, and post-registration education and practice.

Only applications from overseas first-level registered nurses can be accepted by the NMC for registration in the UK, and therefore the following qualifications are not accepted:

- Enrolled nurse
- Licensed practical nurse
- Vocational nurse
- Community nurse
- State certified nurse
- Staff nurse (South Africa)
- Mothercraft nurse
- Nursery nurse.

Although somewhat divorced from the contents of this chapter, it is worth reminding the reader that overseas applicants will also need to meet immigration requirements, and this must be done independently of the NMC.

As well as demonstrating their competence in order to access the NMC register, the applicant must also be able to demonstrate an ability to communicate effectively with patients in English. Unless their exams and training were undertaken in English and English is the language they use for general conversation, they will be expected to gain a threshold mark in the International English Testing System. Note that this rule cannot be applied to applicants from the EU.

When making the decision based on evidence submitted to the NMC there are a number of possible outcomes, namely:

- Accepted for registration

- Required to undertake further education in the UK to develop specified skills and provide reference(s) supporting the application for registration

- Required to undertake a period of practice to prepare for nursing in the UK, and then to provide a reference from the person supervising their practice supporting the application for registration

- Required to provide further information about their education and/or practice

- Rejected if their education and training was not at least 3 years in duration, or if the applicant does not meet the minimum requirements for application.

In some cases you will be the registered nurse who supports and assesses the overseas applicant in relation to their competence in identified areas, and provides, with the support of your manager, the reference to the NMC.

As already suggested, overseas recruitment may be only a short-term solution to the long-term problems of recruitment and retention. The government states that 'by 2004, on current plans, we expect more than 45 000 new nurses and midwives to come out of training' (DoH 2000a, p. 51), and predict that 'as a result of this NHS Plan there will be 5500 more nurses, midwives and health visitors being trained each year by 2004, than today' (DoH 2000a, p. 51).

This recruitment agenda has a major impact upon pre- and post-registration education and training scenarios, namely:

- Do we have the necessary physical resources, in both university and service delivery areas, to support these learners?

● Do we have the necessary human resources to teach and support these learners wherever learning takes place? These human resources include nurse lecturers based and employed in the higher education sector, and registered nurses and midwives in all areas of practice who are vital to teach, assess and support these learners, while at the same time delivering patient care in whatever context they are employed.

Consider these issues and apply them to your own workplace and to your own working practices, as they will affect your ability to practise as an assessor and teacher, as well as a practitioner in health care.

Through whatever route registered nurses come into the health sector, they will all require teaching, support and assessment throughout their various learning pathways. These roles will fall within your remit, supported by other staff, perhaps based in your partner university.

---

**ACTIVITY 2.3**

List all of the staff you think will be included in the teaching, supporting and assessing of nurses in your area.
   You may have listed:

■ All registered nurses
■ Practice educators/facilitators
■ Lecturers
■ Link teachers
■ Other professionals, e.g. physiotherapists.

---

**ACTIVITY 2.4**

List all of the learners you may be involved in teaching and supporting. Your list may include:

■ HCAs
■ Nursing students
■ Second-level nurses undertaking conversion courses
■ First-level nurses undertaking a second branch programme, e.g. mental health nurse working towards adult branch qualification
■ 'Return to practice' nurses – nurse returners
■ Overseas nurses undertaking supervised practice/adaptation programmes
■ Other professional students, e.g. physiotherapy, medicine
■ Other non-professional students, e.g. physiotherapy assistants.

---

As we can see from the above, your teaching skills are needed across a wide range of learners. Perhaps we need to pause here and look at the education and training pathways and processes that might ultimately lead to the development of registered nurses in the first instance.

## HCAS

Most health care employers employ non-professional staff to support professionals – and nursing is no exception. Please note that we do not use the term 'unqualified', as many of these staff have relevant care qualifications in the form of National or Scottish Vocational Qualifications (NVQ/SVQ). It appears that more and more employers are either expecting their non-professional staff to have these qualifications in order to gain employment, or state that the acquisition of such an award within a specific timeframe is a prerequisite of employment. Indeed, the NHS pay modernisation agenda includes a competence framework, known as the Knowledge and Skills Framework (KSF) (see Chapter 4), that will affect *all* NHS staff, regardless of job title or role, professional or non-professional status. Within the KSF the competencies are linked to other nationally accredited competence frameworks, and NVQs and SVQs are included in this. Note that the KSF will be a mandatory framework across the NHS, demonstrating the need for competent staff across the whole employment spectrum.

Both the government and the NMC have recognised the need to value and develop staff with non-professional qualifications, and to credit these staff with previous learning through an accreditation route. In theory this means that a HCA applying for a place on a pre-registration nursing programme, who already has clinical experience and an NVQ level 3 in Care, may undertake a shortened programme, as her experience and qualification are matched against the outcomes of the 3-year pre-registration programme. This is clarified by the UKCC Education Commission's work in 1998, reviewing nursing and midwifery education, where it states that: 'we propose introducing greater flexibility in pre-registration nursing programmes to improve recruitment and retention' (UKCC 1998, p. 27, 3.39). This is taken further as the Commission goes on to recommend the introduction of accreditation of prior experience and learning (AP(E)L), which will then demand the 'restructuring and redesigning for pre-registration programmes to accommodate the effects of these changes and to allow for more flexible progression'.

In practice this has been slow to develop, although there are examples of such developments throughout the UK.

| ACTIVITY 2.5 | Find out if your partner university gives credit for NVQs/SVQs and/or other qualifications into the pre-registration nursing programmes. |
|---|---|

However, before we move into the content and delivery of pre-registration nursing programmes it is necessary to explore the processes of NVQs and SVQs.

# NVQ/SVQ – the background

SVQs/NVQs in Health and Social Care areas were first developed in the late 1980s as a response to the need to educate, train and develop the non-professional workforce employed in these sectors. Since spring 2003, the Sector Skills Council, Skills For Health, has been the official organisation developing NVQs and SVQs for use throughout and within the entire health sector, across all roles, and these qualifications include those developed for HCAs.

Briefly, NVQs and SVQs are qualifications developed by a sector, e.g. health, for a sector, e.g. the vast healthcare sector – which includes public, private and independent sections.

# The NVQ/SVQ framework

It is stated by the Qualifications and Curriculum Authority (QCA) that the NVQ framework 'provides a comprehensive, coherent and transparent national system which indicates the relationship between NVQs at different levels of achievement'. It makes explicit the opportunities for progression and transfer between both qualifications and areas of competence.

SVQs/NVQs are awarded at five different levels and the level descriptors are intended to be indicative rather than prescriptive. It should also be noted that the levels apply to the qualification as a whole and not to the individual units within a qualification. Employers, and indeed practitioners, acting as teachers and assessors of these staff and qualifications, find the definitions of the levels useful in clarifying the status and developmental needs of individuals undertaking awards, especially those in employment. Not all levels apply to each sector, so, for example, the care sector awards cover levels 2, 3 and 4, whereas management awards cover levels 3, 4 and 5.

# Definitions of levels

### LEVEL 1

Competence, which involves the application of knowledge in the performance of a range of varied work activities, most of which may be routine and predictable.

### LEVEL 2

Competence, which involves the application of knowledge in a significant range of varied work activities performed in a variety of contexts. Some of the activities are complex or non-routine, and there is some individual responsibility or autonomy. Collaboration with others, perhaps through membership of a work-group or team, may often be a requirement.

## LEVEL 3

Competence, which involves the application of knowledge in a broad range of work activities, performed in a wide variety of contexts, most of which are complex and non-routine. There is considerable responsibility and autonomy, and responsibility for the work of others may be required.

## LEVEL 4

Competence, which involves the application of knowledge in a broad range of complex, technical or professional activities, performed in a wide variety of contexts and with a substantial degree of personal responsibility and autonomy. There is often responsibility for the work of others and the allocation of resources.

## LEVEL 5

Competence, which involves the application of a significant range of fundamental principles across a wide and often unpredictable variety of contexts. Very substantial personal autonomy and often significant responsibility for the work of others and for the allocation of substantial resources feature strongly, as do personal accountabilities for analysis and diagnosis, design, planning, execution and evaluation (QCA 1997).

Although the competence framework involved within NVQs and SVQs will be looked at in more detail in Chapter 3, it is worth introducing an overview of these awards here so that you can examine the links and progressions from these qualifications to registered nurse status.

NVQs and SVQs are vocational qualifications that are based on and assessed in practice. This does not mean, however, that only practice is assessed, as NVQs/SVQs demand the rigorous assessment of theory, which in turn is applied to practice. This means that the theory–practice gap is filled, as knowledge and practice are assessed in the context of care delivery and not in isolation – and competence is not acknowledged until both parts of the award have been achieved.

The Department of Health (DoH) suggested that a career framework will be developed in the context of career modernisation, and this framework demonstrates a career trajectory from HCA to consultant practitioner (DoH 1999, p. 32) – in the context of nursing, this means consultant nurses (Fig. 2.1).

| **FIGURE 2.1** | *A career framework* |
| --- | --- |

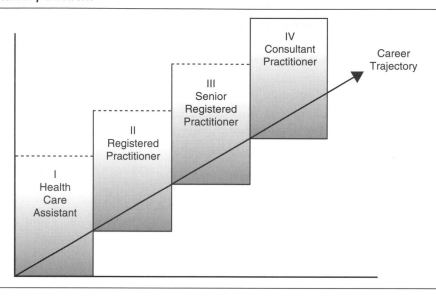

As previously stated, NVQs and SVQs are not mandatory qualifications in the NHS, although there are mandates within the independent sector, especially related to nursing home staff, that do state the target achievement of NVQs to be at least level 2 for 50% of staff by 2004.

Having said that there is no mandate for the achievement of NVQs/SVQs in the NHS, there are developments which imply that these awards are to be valued and encouraged for non-professional staff. Two of these developments are the pay award implemented in April 2002, whereby new pay scales for staff with NVQ levels 2 and 3 were identified at the top of Whitley Grades A and B, and this will be superseded by the pay modernisation (Agenda for Change) implementation due to be launched across the whole of the NHS in 2004. This will be looked at in more detail in Chapter 4.

There is more detail about NVQ/SVQ awards, qualifications and processes in Chapter 3.

## LEARNING IN HIGHER EDUCATION

The movement of all nursing education programmes from Colleges of Nursing, Midwifery and Health Visiting to universities was completed in 1997. This afforded many challenges to the profession, particularly regarding the management of the tensions between research and teaching (both key elements in academia) and providing a clinically credible experience for students (Council of Deans 1999). Alongside this, vocational education has been viewed by some commentators as not having the appropriate academic standing (Floud 2002); consequently, much effort has gone into developing processes that award practice the same standing as academic learning.

The move of nursing education into higher education has required the profession to adopt the systems used within the sector, and as a result it has benefited from the shared learning and transferability that the systems afford. 'Nursing midwifery and health visitor education must continue to be fully integrated within higher education and must enjoy a status equivalent to that of other university students. This implies that the same opportunities for development, including the establishment of links with other subject areas and the pursuit of research, are equal to other disciplines' (National Assembly for Wales 2001, p. 17).

## The necessity for academic rigour

**ACTIVITY 2.6**

In relation to the profession of nursing and midwifery there are many reasons why the processes used in higher education need to be rigorous. Make a list of the reasons why you think it necessary, for both yourself as a teacher, your students and the higher education system in general.

Your answers may include some of the following.
For the teacher:

- To make sure that your teaching meets the required quality standards set by the university and the professional organisation issuing the award

- To make sure that your teaching method will achieve what you want your students to learn. For example, telling students what informed consent is about will not elicit their feelings on the subject or change attitudes (see Chapter 3)

- To diagnose students' strengths, areas where they need to develop and gaps in their learning, in order that remedial action can be taken

- To help you to improve your performance and to improve the conditions for learning by providing feedback.

For the student:

- To be confident that the knowledge acquired is of the same quality and at the same level as that of other students undertaking similar courses

- To provide the opportunity to transfer what has already been learned to another university
- To offer the opportunity to use the learning acquired as part of an application for accreditation towards another course.

For the university system:

- Patient/client safety needs to be at the top of the list. If courses are to be passed successfully, the institution is responsible for ensuring that the award meets any criteria set for public safety. In nursing and midwifery these are set down by the NMC and will be discussed later in this chapter
- To make sure that the systems in place meet the requirements of the agencies charged with monitoring academic standards.

## Academic levels

In general terms higher education pitches its programmes of study on three levels. Academic level 1 is equivalent to certificate level. An example of nurses educated to certificate level are those who undertook their training prior to the inception of Project 2000 courses in the 1980s. Academic level 2 equates to a diploma (in nursing or health studies, for example), and level 3 equates with a degree (for example BSc in Nursing).

## System of accreditation used in higher education

Higher education institutions operate what is known as a credit accumulation and transfer scheme, or CATS for short. This is the system used for awarding credit on study that has been undertaken at the levels identified above. The positive benefit of a CATS system is that it enables the student to obtain some exemption towards a qualification or award by gaining credit for different courses of study and areas of learning that have already been undertaken successfully. This means that the number of credits acquired during the pre-registration programme may be used as 'currency' towards another course.

## PRE-REGISTRATION NURSE EDUCATION PROGRAMMES

All pre-registration nursing education programmes are delivered through partnerships between higher education institutions and service providers, usually in the guise of NHS Trusts. The entry criteria to pre-registration programmes have, historically, been set by the UKCC. More recently, universities have the autonomy to set their own entry criteria, depending on the academic level of the programme, for example diploma or degree, and the need to widen the entry gate to nursing to applicants from non-traditional backgrounds, usually those without accepted educational qualifications in the form of GCSE or A levels. This is in response to the Government's modernisation agenda and is supported by the UKCC document *Fitness for Practice*, which also identified 'the need to offer flexible entry to nursing programmes to attract more recruits with a wider range of skills and abilities into the profession' (UKCC 1998, p. 25, 3.24).

In England pre-registration programmes in nursing are delivered at a variety of academic levels, ranging from diploma, advanced diploma to degree. Successful achievement at any of the above levels will enable the individual to register with the NMC and to work as a registered nurse in environments of their choosing. Scotland, Northern Ireland and Wales have made commitments towards an all degree level pre-registration preparation. There are many issues regarding the varied academic level of the programmes, often linked to financial implications for the students themselves, which may ultimately influence their choice of academic programme.

## Programme content

Regardless of their academic level all programmes enable the students to become registered nurses and to gain employment in such a capacity. All programmes must entail 4600 hours (or 3 years) of learning, 50% of which must be based in practice which 'must be transparent' (UKCC 2001a, p. 5, 1.2).

In the context of a 3-year programme the first year is known as the Common Foundation Programme (CFP), and is common across the current four branches of the programme, namely adult nursing, mental health nursing, learning disability nursing and children's nursing. The next 2 years are branch specific, where knowledge and theory are both applied to the chosen branch of nursing. Exposure to, and placements in, practice areas relevant to the stage of the programme are undertaken at an early stage in the programme, enabling students to develop and apply skills and knowledge as soon as possible, including such skills as communications, as well as the more practical skills such as baseline observations or wound dressing.

As stated earlier in this chapter, some universities will give credit for prior experience and learned knowledge, and students may be seen to undertake a shortened CFP, although when APEL is applied it can be demonstrated that the full 4600 hours have been undertaken.

All pre-registration nurse education is delivered in partnership with universities and NHS Trusts and other service providers. As such, universities develop curricula that meet the requirements of the NMC, but which also are responsive to local needs and demands. It can be seen therefore that no two curricula are exactly the same, although there are common strands throughout all curricula, which leads to the development of registered nurses who can work anywhere within the UK and EU. Their learning will have equipped them with transferable skills and knowledge, and the ability to transfer those skills and knowledge across employment areas and across client groups.

We can consider next the work of the UKCC – now the NMC – which led to the development of outcomes and competencies across the pre-registration programmes, regardless of branch. In this context the UKCC defined competence as 'the skills and ability to practise safely and effectively without the need for direct supervision' (UKCC 1998).

To set this development in context, the Nurses, Midwives and Health Visitors Act 1997 (Section 2(3)) requires the NMC, through rules, to determine the standard, kind and content of training to be undertaken with a view to registration. As already stated, this does not mean that the NMC has developed the curricula for all pre-registration programmes, but the universities develop their own curricula adhering to the rules laid down by the NMC. The UKCC states that 'pre-registration nursing programmes should be designed to prepare the student to be able, on registration, to apply knowledge and understanding and skills when performing to the standards required in employment and to provide the nursing care which patients and clients require, safely and competently, and so assume the responsibilities and accountabilities necessary for public protection' (UKCC 2001c, p. 9:37).

As already discussed, the progammes comprise a 1-year CFP and a 2-year branch programme. The UKCC stated that 'the primary aim in pre-registration nursing programmes is to ensure that students are prepared to practise safely and effectively to such an extent that the protection of the public is assured' (UKCC 2001c, p. 5:16). It is therefore implicit and vital that pre-registration programmes are practice-centred; hence the need for 50% of practice to be transparent in all programmes, building on and supporting the 50% theory contained within the same programme. The ultimate aim is the development of professional competence.

The UKCC recognised that 'safe and effective practice requires a sound underpinning of the theoretical knowledge which informs practice. Such knowledge must therefore be directly related to and integrated within practice' (UKCC 2001c, p. 5:17).

This is where you have a major impact upon students' learning and application, i.e. theory to practice. Most curricula, and the learning that students undertake, introduce the theories and knowledge-base before exposing the students to the applied practice. You, as the teacher in the practice setting, need to be aware of the learning processes of your students, and where they are in relation to their learning. You will then need to enable your students to explore their knowledge, link it to their practice, and consolidate learning. This you can do through devising assessment plans or learning contracts with your students, making the most of all opportunities that present (see supporting learning in practice later in this chapter).

## Outcomes and competencies

The UKCC developed **outcomes** to be achieved within the CFP and **competencies** to be achieved within the branch programme. No student is allowed to progress into their selected branch until they have successfully achieved all of the CFP outcomes, and this includes all areas covered by their practice and theory assessments and assignments.

Domains cover broad areas of practice, though the key descriptors of the domains and their content change as a student moves from CFP to branch programme.

The domains are:

- Professional and ethical practice

- Care delivery

- Care management

- Personal and professional development.

---

**ACTIVITY 2.7**

Compare these domains with the dimensions contained in the KSF in Chapter 4. It is probably helpful here to give you some indication of the detail of some of these domains, both as outcomes and as competencies. However, it is vital that you have a copy of the whole NMC document so that you can become familiar with it and subsequently have a greater understanding of your students' progress and learning needs.

**Domain – Professional and ethical practice**

**Outcome** – Discuss in an informed manner the implications of professional regulation for nursing practice.

**Competence** – Manage oneself, one's practice, and that of others, in accordance with the NMC's *Code of professional conduct*, recognising one's own abilities and limitations.

**Domain – Care delivery**

**Outcome** – Contribute to the development and documentation of nursing assessments by participating in comprehensive and systematic nursing assessment of the physical, psychological, social and spiritual needs of patients and clients.

**Competence** – Undertake and document a comprehensive, systematic and accurate nursing assessment of the physical, psychological, social and spiritual needs of patients, clients and communities.

**Domain – Care management**

**Outcome** – Demonstrate literacy, numeracy and computer skills needed to enter, store, retrieve and organise data essential for care delivery.

**Competence** – Demonstrate key skills in literacy, numeracy, information technology and management and problem solving.

**Domain – Personal and professional development**

**Outcome** – demonstrate responsibility for one's own learning through the development of a portfolio of practice, and recognise when further learning is required.

**Competence** – Demonstrate a commitment to the need for continuing professional development (CPD) and personal supervision activities in order to enhance knowledge, skills, values and attitudes for safe and effective nursing practice.

---

**ACTIVITY 2.8**

Examine the 2001 UKCC document *Requirements for Pre-Registration Nursing Programmes* and compare the outcomes and domains with the units of competence contained in NVQs/SVQs at levels 2 and 3 in Care (Chapter 4), and also the dimensions contained within the KSF (Chapter 4).

You may notice similarities in areas such as:

■ Communication
■ Personal and people development
■ Assessment of health and wellbeing needs
■ and others…

---

As has been identified throughout this chapter and by you the reader, there is commonality across numerous areas of learning, most of which need to be evidenced in portfolios of different kinds. However, because of the similarities it is possible to develop a portfolio of learning that meets all demands and truly fits the lifelong learning agenda of all professional – and a large number of non-professional – staff within and across the whole health sector. Portfolio development is covered in Part 2 of this chapter and in Chapter 4, linked to personal development plans.

## CPD AND LIFELONG LEARNING

Learners of all kinds in the health sector – in particular registered nurses and non-professional carers – need not only to maintain their knowledge and skills gained through practice and formal learning, but also to demonstrate that maintenance. There is also the need to demonstrate the advancement of knowledge and skills in certain areas, identified and agreed between an individual and his or her manager in terms of the NHS KSF (see Chapter 4) and as identified by the individual in relation to personal development.

Although this is not a new process its importance and relevance have been strengthened by the introduction of PREP (The Post-Registration Education and Practice Report) for registered nurses by the UKCC in 1995, and the publication of *Working Together – Learning Together: A Framework for Lifelong Learning in the NHS* (DoH 2001).

PREP applies only to those staff whose names appear on the NMC register, but lifelong learning is rapidly becoming the domain of all professionals and of a substantial number of non-professional and ancillary staff. The DoH states that 'lifelong learning and development are key to delivering the government's vision of patient-centred care in the NHS' (DoH 2001, p. vii). This document goes on to say that the government's aim is to develop and equip staff with the skills they need to:

- Support changes and improvements in patient care

- Take advantage of wider career opportunities

- Realise their potential.

The ideals in this document link to the content of the NHS Plan, and it notes that 'the NHS Plan sets out a radical agenda for modernising education and training' (DoH 2001, p. 1).

A current proposal that might go some way towards meeting this agenda is the Skills Escalator. The government stresses its desire to open up learning opportunities for all staff who join NHS organisations, and the Skills Escalator will provide this. Much of this work is contained within the *Agenda for Change*, focusing on the pay modernisation proposals, and has culminated in the development of:

- An NHS job evaluation scheme to assure the skills and knowledge required for a job

- An NHS KSF (see Chapter 4) which sets out more clearly the competencies required at different stages of career progression for all staff.

These developments put CPD within the scope and expectation of all staff.

Another focus in the document is that of increased interprofessional education, and suggests that 'there should be core skill elements in learning programmes for all health professional students, which provide the basis for common and interprofessional learning' (DoH 2001, p. 26). A number of universities are developing shared learning, often classroom based, but there are also developments to expand this to practice settings, the intention being to attempt to breakdown professional barriers and, some would argue, professional tribalism. This will be addressed in the next chapter.

Throughout this chapter most of the content has concerned the literature and processes that support and develop learning, and has yet to cover the practical issues of how you support and teach learners in practice.

The first step will be for you to find out which programme your student is undertaking, and then to find out where they are currently placed within that programme. For a student nurse you might find that they have completed their CFP and have just embarked upon their branch programme. Your clinical area is their first placement within this part of their programme.

You may be supporting an HCA who is undertaking a NVQ level 3 in Care, having already successfully achieved a level 2. As an HCA she is likely to be a permanent member of your staff, and you may well be her named assessor. As an NVQ assessor you will be aware of the need of the assessment process to assess knowledge alongside practice – and to assess both as part of care. You will know which units the HCA has completed and which are to be taught and assessed.

Once you have identified the programme and the stage of learning the student is now undertaking, you will need to clarify and utilise prior learning so as to move into new areas, while at the same time enabling the student to consolidate learning that has already taken place.

From this point you need to develop with your student a learning contract, according to the curriculum they are working to, and to the programme and individual learning objectives that the student identifies as necessary to this part of their learning programme. Remember it is no use asking the learner what they want to learn if they don't know what's on offer: your care environment may be a very new experience for them. You therefore need to highlight the learning opportunities that present themselves in your area, and allow the student to be exposed to such situations.

So, let's list your processes for successful learning and teaching:

- Identify what programme of study your student is undertaking

- Identify how far your student has progressed in the programme

- Identify and utilise any prior learning

- Devise a learning contract with your student.

# PART 2: THE LEARNING AND TEACHING JOURNEY: BECOMING AN EXPERT

## PATHWAY TO EXPERT PRACTICE

We start this second part of the chapter with a number of questions, as expertise is a complex subject with many facets.

| ACTIVITY 2.9 | First of all, stop for a moment and consider how you would define an expert. It doesn't have to relate to nursing practice … what about an expert car mechanic, decorator or cook? Now compare your answer with some of the definitions that follow. |
| --- | --- |

The 1996 *Concise Oxford Dictionary* tells us that an expert is 'one who has special skill at a task or knowledge in a subject'. Its root is shared with that of the word 'experience', meaning 'actual observation of or practical acquaintance with facts or events'. So an expert has something to do with knowing and being good at something – and some of that expertise may have been gained by watching and doing things in practice. Note that the dictionary refers to *special* skill or knowledge. We need to recognise that not everyone can become an expert – some people may stop their learning journey before they reach this stage.

Polyani (1958) differentiates between two types of knowing: *knowing that* – that is, knowing about something – knowing the underlying theory, and *knowing how* – which refers to skill or practical knowledge. You can have know-how without the underpinning theory. For instance, you could teach a patient's partner to record blood pressure. However, if they had no underlying theory they would be unable to make sense of, or interpret, what they had found. Nurses need both kinds of knowledge in order to see the whole picture of what is happening to a patient.

A lot of our knowledge about expertise in nursing comes from some seminal descriptive research carried out by Benner (1984) in the early 1980s in California. In her work she researched and then describes the journey – much as we are doing here in this chapter – from novice to expert, frequently using the words of over 1200 nurses who took part in her research.

Benner says that to understand expertise in nursing you have first to look at the knowledge that is embedded in practice. This knowledge was often hidden in the past, because nurses were poor at articulating it or describing it systematically. This meant that nursing often became invisible: if nurses are unable to say what it is they do, then others will not recognise their unique

| BOX 2.1 | *Benner's domains of nursing practice (from Benner 2001, with permission)* |
|---------|---------------------------------------------------------------------------|

- The helping role
- The teaching–coaching function
- The diagnostic and patient monitoring function
- Effective management of rapidly changing situations
- Administering and monitoring therapeutic interventions and regimens
- Monitoring and ensuring the quality of health care practices
- Organisational and work-role competencies.

contribution. In exploring how expertise develops over time, Benner looked at how nurses made decisions in seven domains of nursing practice (Box 2.1).

| ACTIVITY 2.10 | Now think about an expert nurse that you know. What is it about him or her that is different from a newly registered practitioner? How would you recognise expertise in practice? |
|---------------|---|

Benner would say that an expert nurse is able to recognise quite subtle changes in a patient's condition, using their past experiences in other situations to guide their present actions and perceptions. As an example, a competent registered practitioner would know what to do if a patient had a haematemesis, whereas an expert nurse would anticipate the haematemesis, spotting the signs and symptoms of it before it occurred. He or she, having experienced this situation in the past, might use intuition to guide their actions. All registered nurses would anticipate bleeding if the patient's heart rate rose and blood pressure fell – but the expert might get a feel for – and anticipate – bleeding even while the blood pressure was still within normal limits, perhaps by noticing increased restlessness or a change in skin colour. They can, in this way, act as an early warning system for other health care professionals, as they are constantly with the patient.

An expert, therefore, is not bound by rules and can take informed risks. The point here, though, is that the risks are informed by both learned theory and rich experience. Experts use this blend of formal learning and experience to help them to manage complex situations.

A key facet of expertise is what it brings to the patient. An expert can help a patient – and his or her carers – to gain a sense of control over the situation, coaching them through their illness and educating them along their healthcare journey.

All the above, then, are facets of expertise. If you are reading this book we assume that you have a particular interest in learning and teaching, and so it is worth exploring further what Benner (2001) has to say in Chapter 5 of *From Novice to Expert*, which examines the domain of the teaching–coaching function. She identifies a number of interventions that expert

| BOX 2.2 | *Benner's competencies of the expert nurse in the teaching and coaching domain of practice (from Benner 2001, with permission)* |
|---------|---------------------------------------------------------------|
| | ■ Timing: capturing a patient's readiness to learn – and his or her receptiveness to information<br>■ Assisting patients to integrate the implications of illness and recovery into their lifestyles – maximising abilities and coping with disabilities<br>■ Eliciting and understanding the patient's interpretation of his or her illness – and respecting this<br>■ Providing an interpretation of the patient's condition and explaining why particular treatments and care have been planned, in words that the patient can understand<br>■ The coaching function – helping the patient understand and cope with uncharted and painful experiences – being there for the patient on his or her journey. |

nurses make in relation to educating patients about their illness/health journey – and easing their way along that path. These include:

- Forewarning patients about what to expect and ensuring that they have the correct information to help them to understand and cope with what is happening to them

- Taking 'what is foreign and fearful to the patient and making it familiar and thus less frightening' (p. 77)

- Communicating effectively 'in extreme circumstances' with someone who is ill and frightened

- Responding to the individual patient and his or her circumstances. There is no set pattern or recipe and we cannot generalise about what works. Each person and his or her life and health situation is unique: humour may work for some patients but not for others; authoritative tones may sometimes be what is needed; equally, acting for the patient, rather than expecting self-care, may sometimes be appropriate.

Box 2.2 shows Benner's competencies of the expert nurse in the teaching and coaching domain of practice.

| ACTIVITY 2.11 | Get hold of a copy of Benner's classic work *From Novice to Expert* and read at least Chapter 5 – although the whole book is well worth reading. In this chapter she gives lots of practice examples which will bring her work alive for you.<br>    Now think of a nurse in your own clinical area whom you consider to be an expert practitioner and ask if you can shadow him or her for an hour, when s/he is talking to patients in his or her care. Look at the competencies of the expert nurse in the teaching–coaching domain in Box 2.2 and try to find concrete |

practice examples of how your expert demonstrated each competency. Find some time to discuss these with him or her, and ask how they developed these skills over time.

You may find that your expert finds it hard to articulate exactly how they developed the skills, seeing it as something that happened imperceptibly, with experience. The journey from novice to expert, in the past, has been infrequently recorded, with few points on the map documented. In future, now that health professionals keep portfolios we should be better at describing how we arrive at the point of expertise, although it is doubtful if most experts would describe themselves as such!

Benner defines the stages in the journey as:

- **Novice** – a beginner with no experience and little understanding, but with some theoretical (textbook) and rule knowledge. Note than an experienced nurse can become a novice for a while when entering a new milieu. Behaviour cannot adapt to differing individuals and contexts and is rule bound. This can be referred to as the stage of 'unconscious incompetence'.

- **Advanced beginner** – someone who can demonstrate acceptable performance, using rote behaviour with limited personal experience. This person needs support and guidance for actions and priority setting, as a result of paucity of professional experience. They are starting to work out patterns in the experience that they have had – the stage of 'conscious incompetence'.

- **Competent** – a practitioner who has probably been in his or her area of clinical practice for 2–3 years, who can see which aspects of the patient journey are crucial and which are less so, and who can set priorities accordingly. This nurse is starting to feel that he or she can manage what is going on. Planning is conscious and deliberate – this is the stage of 'conscious competence'.

- **Proficient** – now the nurse sees situations in the round, rather than as a series of separate tasks that have to be performed. They can see the longer-term goals in a situation and are beginning to use experience to foretell what might happen in a given scenario. They know what might be expected to happen and what aspects of a situation might be the most important and telling. They can home in on what aspects are key.

- **Expert** – this practitioner no longer relies on rules or principles to guide behaviour: he or she has an 'intuitive grasp of each situation and zeroes in on the accurate region of the problem without wasteful consideration of a large range of unfruitful, alternative diagnoses and solutions' (p. 32).

Like the chess master, the expert nurse cannot always articulate why he or she has done something ... the expert might say it just felt right – and this results from plentiful and rich experience in a range of similar situations. Here the practitioner is 'unconsciously competent' – care is fluid and seamless and highly effective, and is delivered seemingly without undue conscious effort.

So what does experience mean? It does not mean simply working for a long time in a particular specialism; rather, it refers to working with lots of similar situations which add shades of opinion; it depends on practising in a specialism for a long enough time to ask pertinent questions; to interpret similar situations differently according to their context; and to attempt potentially risky behaviour in a bid to solve a patient's problem.

Not all nurses, however, take Benner's perspective. Conway (1996), for example, takes a stance based in the UK (rather than the USA). She examined the knowledge used by the expert nurse, arguing that this demonstrates the evolution of the expert nurse in the UK. In her research she divided expert nurses into four groups according to their exhibited characteristics:

- **Technologists** – those who demonstrated a range of knowledge and who were able to diagnose – in effect, those who were able to use a lot of the knowledge used by medical colleagues

- **Traditionalists** – practitioners who were concerned with accomplishing the job; care was based on a medical model and practitioners acted as doctors' assistants. Nurses did not value their own practice and education was extra to requirements. There was no value attached to reflection

- **Specialists** – these practitioners varied in what they did within their specialisms. Some prescribed treatments; all were extending the roles of nurses. Some were prescribing drugs; some were undertaking the tasks of doctors

- **Humanistic existentialists** – these were practitioners with a recognisable focus on holistic nursing; they were focused exclusively on nursing practice and its development. Practitioners were prepared to take risks and saw themselves as leaders in their practice arena.

**ACTIVITY 2.12**   Read both Benner's and Conway's differentiations of expertise again. Try to see where these classifications differ: they both describe a journey towards expertise. Which one do you feel most comfortable with?

There is no right or wrong answer here. By the end of this section it would be good if you could find a framework to describe the acquisition of expertise that you feel happy with in your own practice.

Higgs and Titchen (2001) come at expertise from a different direction again, exploring what professional practice knowledge is and how it underpins expertise and its development. Expertise derives from a synthesis of knowledge that comes from theory and research, personal knowledge and professional knowledge.

Knowledge that comes from theory, scholarship and research is called **propositional knowledge**. It is formal and based on relationships – e.g. between cause and effect; usually it is regarded as transferable knowledge. It has long been applied to underpin the practice of professionals.

However, practice is not simple. Professionals – nurses – work in an area where problems are not straightforward: they are complex and based on uncertain ground; bound up with the intimate and personal details of the clients and patients for whom they care – and their families. This is what Schon (1987) referred to as the 'swampy lowlands' of professional practice: seeing practice as messy and ambiguous, and requiring constant adjustments in order to solve problems.

Propositional knowledge mixes here with **personal** knowledge – knowledge that comes from life experience; self-awareness; knowledge about 'what makes people tick'; knowledge that can be used to help interpret what lies behind the spoken or unspoken words of patients and clients.

**Professional craft knowledge** develops over time, with experience of nursing practice. It is a blend of knowing what has happened in the past in other similar scenarios and knowing what worked then, and knowing this particular patient/client now. From all this, together with an understanding of the underpinning theory, the nurse can select from his or her practice repertoire of actions to plan, deliver and evaluate care.

Expertise results from the ways in which nurses use this blend of the three types of knowledge within practice.

**ACTIVITY 2.13**

Think of how you solved a problem in a patient's care sometime in the last week. Can you identify the three sorts of knowledge that you might have used, as a mix, in forming a solution? What was the underpinning theory/research? What personal life experience or knowledge did you use? What did you draw on from your past professional practice?

In future, when you are reflecting on what you did well or could have done better at the end of a shift, try to think about the knowledge that you used and how you blended it.

Manley and McCormack (1997) described the five key attributes of the expert nurse, based on Benner's work, as:

1. **Holistic practice knowledge**   This refers to using a blend of different types of knowledge in order to offer the best possible 'all-round'

(holistic) care, being mindful of the patient's – and his or her family's – physical, social, psychological and spiritual needs.

2. **Saliency**   Quite simply, this means knowing which is the right thing to do when; being able to pick out which are the most important things to attend to in a practice situation; being able to home in on priorities in this particular patient, at this particular time.

3. **Knowing the patient**   This means having taken the trouble to get to know him or her as a person; knowing how he or she will respond in all of the domains referred to above. Experts need to know this in order to plan effective care.

4. **Moral agency**   This is to do with respecting the patient; affording them dignity, protecting them and acting as their advocate when they are vulnerable; helping the patient (and their family) to feel safe; offering comfort; and at all times maintaining integrity in the nurse–patient relationship.

5. **Skilled know-how**   Delivering nursing care of the highest standard, seamlessly and apparently effortlessly. This is the stage of unconscious competence referred to earlier in relation to Benner's expert nurse, where the nurse is attuned to the patient in every way.

Manley and McCormack support this by saying that the factors that enable these five attributes of expertise are:

- An ability to reflect on one's practice
- Being authoritative about one's practice and accepting accountability for what one does in practice
- Having a therapeutic relationship with both other team members and patients – using oneself as a person
- Taking a person-centred approach to care delivery – valuing and respecting the patient as a person who has both choice and autonomy.

This chapter is all about supporting the learning journey. In the last few sections we have been looking at the practitioner's journey towards expertise. In some ways it might seem quite strange to be talking still about the practitioner as a learner, when clearly he or she is registered as they move towards expertise. This is something that we will look at in more detail in the next section, where we will focus on lifelong learning – and where we are always learners from the cradle to the grave!

This also implies that practitioners as teachers are never out of a job! They are not concerned simply with supporting the journey to registration, but also with helping to develop the attributes of expertise in themselves and in those with whom they work. In fact, it is a fairly seamless journey, where there are just a few touchdowns for refuelling – registration is one of these stopping points.

---

**ACTIVITY 2.14**

Using one of Manley and McCormack's enabling factors – reflection – think back on your last shift and think when and how you used each of the attributes of expertise. Look back at the explanations now to remind yourself of what they mean. Remembering the underlying meaning may be more helpful that trying to remember words like 'saliency'.

Were you surprised at how you demonstrated each of them in your own practice? You might not yet have come to see yourself as an expert, but perhaps you can now see expertise growing in your practice? Try this exercise from time to time and you will see how your skills develop incrementally. Celebrate this!

So is this what is called lifelong learning? What does that mean?

---

## THE CONCEPT OF LIFELONG LEARNING

Lifelong learning is the term often used to refer to the learning that occurs throughout the – usually working – life of an individual, which may be planned or not. Increasingly, in further and higher education in the UK, learning arising from experience, and reflection in and on practice, has come to be recognised as a valid component of an individual's education, and is given formal recognition in APEL.

The concept of lifelong learning acknowledges that we are in an era of continuous change, and this requires an acceptance that learning occurs at all points in the practitioner's career journey. This implies, of course, that teaching methods appropriate to adult learners must be used, focusing on learning derived from experience, using a student-centred, needs-based approach. This approach – referred to as androgogy (see later) – allows the learner to set his or her own agenda and assess its success. It stresses active, rather than passive, learning, frequently using peers as a source of knowledge.

---

**ACTIVITY 2.15**

For this next week on duty try to make a note of all the new things that you learn in the course of your work.

There may be formal learning opportunities … some things may be learned from caring for patients or speaking with their relatives; multiprofessional colleagues may offer you another perspective on your practice; you may learn from mistakes that you might make – equally from your successes.

The opportunities are there and they are boundless. Capturing and reflecting on some of them like this should help you to see the numerous ways in which you can help other practitioners to share your knowledge and expertise as they learn throughout their careers.

The rapid pace of change in the nature of work today necessitates both planned learning opportunities and valuing the learning that comes from carrying out the job and reflecting on outcomes. 'The growth of knowledge and increasing research in all areas of health care, together with the development of new technology, means that old knowledge and skills are no longer appropriate' (Hinchliff 1994). Lifelong learning is necessary to maintain a skilled workforce in a constantly changing world.

Lifelong learning is associated with values and outcomes, such as:

- Being offered equality of opportunity to learn

- The importance of self-fulfilment

- Having freedom to learn

- Taking responsibility for oneself and one's own learning

- Valuing what other learners can teach

- Having an enquiring mind, able to think critically

- Facilitating others' learning and seeking facilitation for one's own learning.

It refers to a continuum of learning opportunities, from formal teaching to experiential and reflective learning. For lifelong learning to be effective the learner needs to work towards achieving some skills and competencies. Cropley (1981) suggests the following framework:

- **An ability to set and work towards realistic goals that are achievable within the individual's personal and professional life.** This requires a self-directed approach towards learning. Practitioners may need help in setting, and adjusting to, short-, medium- and long-term goals for their own development that are realistic for them. Some learners have a tendency to aim for alpha grades, when beta is more achievable (bearing in mind the demands of, say, a full-time job as a community nurse, two small children, a partner and a home to run, as well as overseeing elderly parents and in-laws, and maintaining some semblance of a social life!).

- **Effective application of theory in practice to tackle work-based problems and an ability to measure the results.** New work-based problems arise as practice constantly develops. For example, with a short inpatient stay people are being discharged home, needing different sorts of care from community nurses from that required in the past. Similarly, with day surgery, nursing care planning has to be adapted to the restricted patient stay, using standard care plans. Practitioners need to be able to reframe in order to look at problems and their solutions in different ways, 'sideways or upside down: to put them in another perspective or another context: to think of them as opportunities not problems' (Handy 1989, p. 52).

- **Maintaining motivation to learn continuously and an ability to evaluate the effectiveness of this learning.** Houle (1980), in his classic work, divided practitioners into five main groups, depending on what he calls their 'zest for learning':
  - innovators: a small but highly active group, who constantly seek to improve their job performance. They try out untested ideas, constantly consume educational opportunities and enjoy independent learning and full time study;
  - pacesetters: not usually the first to try out new ideas, but strongly committed to professional ideals and continuing education;
  - middle majority: the bulk of practitioners, whose attitudes to continuing education vary from enthusiasm to apathy;
  - laggards: those who do the minimum necessary, resisting both learning and new ideas.

Houle also cites a fifth group whom he called facilitators, comprising those who no longer actively practise, consisting of academics, editors, writers and executives, each of whom can fall into any of the preceding four groupings in terms of their motivation towards continuing their education.

- **Familiarity with a variety of learning and assessment strategies in a range of settings ... by definition this demands good study skills and a knowledge of one's own learning style.** If, as stated earlier, adults learn best with an androgogical approach, then the philosophy underlying this may need to be explained, as it may not fit with learners' expectations. Adults tend to learn best when:
  - They experience a 'need to know' and participate voluntarily in the search for knowledge and skills to meet their need;
  - They are in an environment which is both physically and psychologically comfortable, with respect for their own worth and that of others;
  - They are able to set their own goals for their achievements;
  - They share responsibility for both planning and applying their learning;
  - They engage in active rather than passive learning;
  - They are encouraged to relate what they learn to their own experience, and also to use this experience to enrich and inform their learning;

– They feel a sense of responsibility – a sense of ownership – for their own progress.

Although we know that adults learn best when these condition are met, nevertheless, adults who undertook their initial school and nurse education when there was an emphasis on the teacher imparting knowledge to the learner may need space to refocus, learning that it is desirable and permissible to value that which has been derived from experience, to set goals, and to see education as a collaborative partnership between teacher and learner.

- **An ability to locate relevant information and resources, using appropriate media.** If self-direction in learning is to be encouraged throughout the professional's life, then teaching study skills appropriate to this is essential. It is common today for study skills to be taught, not only during schooling, but also as part of pre-registration nurse education. Skills include active reading, listening, problem-solving and decision-making, keyboard and wordprocessing skills, accessing information from databases, online journals, the Internet or library searching etc. There are, however, large numbers of practitioners who were educated before this formed part of the curriculum, and who trained in nursing when these skills were not taught, and so there is considerable unmet need in this area.

**ACTIVITY 2.16**

Having worked through this section, take a few moment to think about the ways in which you learn best. Think about Houle's classification of learners: which category do you think you fall into? Does the above list of factors that help adults to learn apply to you?

There are obviously no right answers here – we each have individual approaches to learning, but it really does help to know the conditions under which you find it easiest to learn.

If we accept that the above are relevant transferable skills and competencies, then CPD should focus on meeting these needs. Lifelong learning embraces the link between education and work – the application of any relevant learning to practice and the notion that practice itself is not static.

Alongside this is the acceptance that theory not only informs a professional's practice, but also that knowledge can be embedded in, and emerge from, practice (Schon 1987). Practice development is underpinned by education that is work focused. Practitioners need to be able to access knowledge and skills and develop attitudes to upgrade – consciously, systematically and continuously – their existing competencies. **CPD** is a way of meeting this need for education 'on the job'.

CPD is the maintenance and enhancement of the knowledge, expertise and competence of professionals throughout their careers according to a plan formulated with regard to the needs of the professional, the employer, the profession and society' (Madden and Mitchell 1993).

It is useful to consider briefly the criteria against which *effective* CPD can be measured:

- The use of a range of strategies to effect learning
- Flexibility in terms of how, where and what the learner learns
- Acceptance of the learning that can accrue from experience and reflection.

Adults have a wealth of experience which they bring to a learning situation and these experiences affect how they perceive their world. They are a rich resource on which to base teaching and learning. Such learning is referred to as **experiential**. If learners are to be encouraged to build on their prior experience, then they may need to be taught to reflect critically upon it.

**Reflection** is the way in which professionals reflect **on** action retrospectively, and also **in** action as it occurs, constantly adjusting practice to 'fit' the cues that are received. Reflective practice recognises the knowledge that is embedded – the tacit knowledge that is the domain of the intuitive expert practitioner, who often knows more than he or she can say. Benner (1984) expands on this in her discussion of expertise in nursing:

Expertise in complex human decision making, such as nursing requires, makes the interpretation of clinical situations possible, and the knowledge embedded in this clinical expertise is central to the advancement of nursing practice and the development of nursing science. Not all the knowledge embedded in expertise can be captured in theoretical propositions' (p. 30).

Cervero (1988) suggests that a culture which fosters lifelong learning encompasses:

- The existence of a positive and valuing attitude within the professional group towards lifelong learning.
- Ensuring that the conditions for learning, and for responding to change, are in tune with the needs of the practitioner, his or her colleagues and the organisation.

One of the conditions for successful uptake of lifelong learning opportunities is what can be referred to as 'felt need'. It is important that it is the potential consumer who perceives this need. Organisational need may well exist, but being sent to learn is ineffective if the learner does not see it as fitting in with his or her own needs.

- Envisaging the need for CPD, and its relevance, right from the stage of initial professional education
- An emphasis on helping practitioners to learn effectively
- The provision of support and guidance for lifelong learners.

This will vary between and within organisations, depending on the pervading management culture. In situations where mentorship or facilitation is valued and continues beyond basic education, and where clinical supervision is seen as a key strategy for developing practice, then such support is likely. Elsewhere support may be patchy, depending on the value managers attach to learning. Even so, peer support can be extremely helpful.

- Seeing people (and investment in them) as an asset to the organisation.

**ACTIVITY 2.17**  So how does the organisation in which you work measure up here? Is it supportive of lifelong learning?
  Even if you think it could do better, you could apply these principles to your immediate workplace and see what you could do to improve the culture there. Take just one item from the list and plan to improve that over the next month.

So far in this chapter we have looked at the journey towards expert practice; lifelong learning; how people learn best; CPD; and fostering an effective culture for learning to occur.

Now we need to think about how this learning can be captured. There will come points in a practitioner's learning and teaching career where he or she needs to provide evidence that they have gained competencies, knowledge, skills – and offer that evidence to others who may measure it against standards of, say, expertise. Equally, as a practice teacher you may be helping other practitioners to do this as part of their lifelong learning journey. This process of measuring evidence against standards or competencies is part of **professional accreditation,** which is discussed in more detail in Chapter 4.

The most usual way of presenting such evidence is in a **professional portfolio**.

# PORTFOLIO DEVELOPMENT (see also Chapter 1)

One of the most commonly used definitions of a portfolio is provided by Brown (1995):

> ... a private collection of evidence which demonstrates the continuing acquisition of skills, knowledge, attitudes, understanding and achievement. It is both retrospective and prospective as well as indicating the current state of development and activity of the individual.

The maintenance of a professional portfolio serves a number of useful purposes, including:

- Valuing yourself and your skills and knowledge, both personally and as a professional
- Keeping a record of professional updating for NMC PREP requirements
- Providing evidence for performance appraisal
- The identification of needs during development reviews
- Aiding career development
- Providing additional insights into your experience for your current or prospective employer
- Demonstrating independent learning
- Encouraging reflective practice
- Providing a permanent record of achievement over time.

Brown sees a **profile** as:

> ... constructed from evidence selected from the personal portfolio for a particular purpose and for the attention of a particular audience.

A portfolio of evidence for accreditation is more than a profile but less than a general personal portfolio of lifelong learning. It is a purposeful collection of evidence that sets out to demonstrate that its holder 'measures up' against the standards or competencies set for the accreditation scheme in question. These standards (usually accompanied by performance criteria) or competencies are determined by experts in the area of clinical practice under consideration. The portfolio of evidence is assessed for sufficiency and rigour by peers. The process of compilation is frequently facilitated and is seen as a developmental opportunity in itself. You may be asked to support another practitioner in this.

The portfolio describes the journey towards the acquisition of the standards, detailing the reflections, insights, knowledge and skills gained along the way. It therefore describes a pathway – often over a period of 1–3 years, which forms a focused part of the overall lifetime career journey.

| ACTIVITY 2.18 | Think how information might be presented to satisfy these two requirements – you are likely to be asked by practitioners to support them in the collection and presentation of such material. |
| --- | --- |

Below are some suggestions to help structure your thoughts and ideas about what a portfolio might look like for accreditation. However, remember that each portfolio will be highly personalised, so that what is relevant information to some practitioners will not be significant or pertinent to the clinical situation, experience or learning of others. If you are supporting practitioners in gathering evidence of their learning you might like to use some of the ideas below. You might also like to try out the methods yourself before you guide others in using them.

## CAPTURING THE EVIDENCE

- **Critical incident reflections**    Write out a reflection on a critical incident that explores a key aspect of your work. Write the reflection in a way that captures the experience and how you dealt with it, who else was involved, perhaps you discussed things with a colleague? Write all this down.
  - Ask yourself questions such as What was it that led you to make the decisions you did?
  - What are the cues that help make explicit what you do everyday in your working life?
  - Where did your insights come from, what triggered your actions, thoughts, feelings?
  - Show your reflection to someone who can offer you some constructive criticisms – they might be able to pick out aspects of your work you had not considered.

- **Direct observation of practice**    Ask your clinical supervisor, facilitator or a colleague to observe you in action. Ask them for annotated notes or reflections to help capture your actions and any outcomes. Then think about how this might become evidence to demonstrate your particular expertise. It can be used to supplement critical reflection of practice.

- **Supervision or action learning notes**    You might also wish to include some evidence of the joint dialogue you have with your colleagues, team, supervisor or facilitator. What has the journey been like in exploring/evaluating/improving clinical practice? How have you managed to find the evidence-base for and/or an increased understanding of your practice? Has this experience filtered through into other work you do? Are there any other people/processes you use that help you critique your work?

- **360° feedback**   You might wish to think about gathering some feedback about your work from nursing colleagues, clients and others in the multidisciplinary team who interface with you. This might include using interviews, testimonials, a questionnaire to a group of people that could be analysed and presented in a portfolio. Try to use people who are familiar with your work who can help you identify aspects of your practice that you have not been able to articulate or identify yourself. This might be through written discussions or even audio tapes.

- **User perspectives**   You might try to get specific user feedback. For instance, you might like to include examples of patients' thank you letters. You may have other organisational systems in place that capture user feedback: think about how you can include these in a portfolio. Remember that if you are using evidence from patients make sure that you have their consent and that confidentiality is not breached. It should not be possible to identify patients from any evidence.

- **Outcomes**   It is important to think about and demonstrate in the portfolio how actions have influenced and affected patient care. Use anything that helps to identify this process. You might have some audit trails that map the process that led to any outcomes. Some questions you can think about are:
  - What and how people are affected by your interactions and interventions?
  - How does practice change in your clinical area?
  - What do peers say about you and your sphere of influence?
  This will all help to enable you to capture and verify your contributions to the workplace.

- **Action learning**   'A continuous process of learning and reflection, supported by colleagues, with the intention of getting things done' (McGill and Beaty 1998).
  You may be part of an action learning set and wish to include some evidence from this process in your portfolio.
  Action learning is an approach to individual and group development, traditionally used to develop managerial and organisational

effectiveness. Over several months, people work in a small group (an action learning set) to tackle important organisational issues or problems and learn from their attempts to change things. Action learning comprises four elements:

- The person – everyone joins and takes part voluntarily
- The problem – everyone brings and must 'own' a problem on which he or she wants to act, in this case an issue to do with the implementation of clinical supervision
- The group or set – because we often need colleagues to help us tackle difficult problems
- The action and the learning – after having analysed the problems, thought through the options and decided what to do, with the help of the set, individuals act to resolve their problems.

Action groups, or action learning sets, meet to help each other think through the issues, create options, agree on action and learn from the effects of that action through providing high challenge and high support. Learning about how groups work is an added benefit. The colleagues in the set may be from the same organisation or from different organisations.

The facilitator's role is to help the set to develop, to facilitate the supporting and challenging processes and to help members reflect on their own learning. The main purpose is to help members towards a deeper understanding of themselves and their practice – and increased effectiveness in their work.

- **Writing narratives**   Finally, you need to build up a clear and convincing discussion of what your evidence demonstrates. Just as a barrister will have to use different pieces of evidence to persuade a jury of the guilt or innocence of a client, you will have to do the same to demonstrate that you have met the standards and competencies in question. It is not sufficient simply to let the evidence speak for itself. You must select your evidence thoughtfully and then link this to particular outcomes, standards or competencies.

**ACTIVITY 2.19**

It is time now to get out your own portfolio and look at the methods you have used to capture evidence of your ability to develop your practice. Have you used all or any of the ways described above? They are not prescriptive, but are cited as a variety of methods that might work for some people. You might like to select a way of exploring practice that you have not used before and try it in your own practice. Once you feel confident in its use you may want to use it in teaching others how to select and present evidence.

# CONCLUSION

In this chapter we have explored the career journey that a practitioner may travel from healthcare assistant to expert nurse. We have focused on this latter stage, examining the steps taken to reach that point. Lifelong learning has been taken as the thread that accompanies the learner from novice to expert. The chapter concluded by detailing the ways in which evidence of learning might be obtained, and how this might be captured in a portfolio.

# REFERENCES

Benner P (ed). From novice to expert: excellence and power in clinical nursing, 2nd edn. California: Pearson Education, 2001

Brown R. Portfolio development and profiling for nurses. Lancaster: Quay Publishing, 1995

Cervero R. Effective continuing education for professionals. San Francisco: Jossey-Bass, 1988

Concise Oxford Dictionary. Oxford: Oxford University Press, 1996

Conway J. Nursing experience and advanced practice. Salisbury: Quay Books, 1996

Council of Deans and Heads of UK University Faculties for Nursing, Midwifery and Health Visiting. Breaking the boundaries: educating nurses, midwives and health visitors for the next millenium. A position paper, 1999

Cropley A. Lifelong learning: a rationale for teacher training. Journal of Education for Teaching 1981; 7

Department of Health. Making a difference. London: The Stationery Office, 1999

Department of Health. The NHS plan – a plan for investment, a plan for reform. London: The Stationery Office, 2000a

Department of Health. A health service for all talents: developing the NHS workforce. London: The Stationery Office, 2000b

Department of Health. Working together – learning together: a framework for lifelong learning for the NHS. London: The Stationery Office, 2001

Floud R. Higher education, the economy and society: developing vocational relevance, 2002 (Available at http://www.universitiesuk. ac.uk/speeches/show.asp?sp=48)

Handy C. The age of unreason. London: Century Business, 1989

Hinchliff S. Learning for life. Nursing Standard 1994; 8: 20–21

Higgs J, Titchen A (eds) Practice knowledge and expertise. Oxford: Butterworth-Heinemann, 2001

Houle C. Continuing learning in the professions. San Francisco: Jossey Bass, 1980

Madden C, Mitchell V. Professions, standards and competence: a survey of continuing education for the professions. Bristol: University of Bristol Department for Continuing Education, 1993

Manley K, McCormack B. Exploring expert practice. MSc Distance Learning module. London: Royal College of Nursing, 1997

McGill I, Beaty L. Action learning. London: Kogan Page, 1998

National Assembly for Wales. Briefing paper 1. Creating the potential: a plan for education, 2001

Polyani M. Personal knowledge. London: Routledge and Kegan Paul, 1958

QCA. Vocational qualifications in England, Wales and Northern Ireland. QCA, 1997

Schon D. The reflective practitioner: how professionals think in action. London: Temple Smith, 1987

UKCC. Fitness for practice – the UKCC commission for nursing and midwifery education. London: UKCC, 1998

UKCC. Fitness for practice and purpose – the report of the UKCC's post commission development group. London: UKCC, 2001a

UKCC. Registering as a nurse or midwife in the United Kingdom – a guide for employers. London: UKCC, 2001b

UKCC. Requirements for pre-registration nursing programmes. London: UKCC, 2001c

# 3 Learning and teaching in practice

*Sue Howard*

- ◆ Providing a structure for teaching
  Aims and objectives
  Identifying what to teach
  Identifying your aim for the session
- ◆ Formal and informal teaching
- ◆ Deciding what to teach
- ◆ Different approaches to teaching
  Creating a good environment for teaching
- ◆ Teaching methods
  Handouts
  Delivering a lecture
  Discussion and tutorial groups
- ◆ Audiovisual aids

## INTRODUCTION

Chapters 1 and 2, in covering issues such as expert practice, higher education, continuing professional development and recruitment and retention, have described learning as being the vehicle through which we develop. Learning is the essential ingredient in the way our future is shaped, either on a personal level or through career development. It is important to look more closely at what learning involves in order to make teaching relevant and effective.

The purpose of this chapter is to explore what is meant by learning and teaching in practice, and to outline the strategies that can be adopted to ensure learning is effective.

### LEARNING OBJECTIVES

After reading this chapter, you should be able to:

- ◆ Discuss the interdependent nature of learning and teaching
- ◆ Recognise the importance of individual differences in the learning process
- ◆ Identify the learning theories that underpin the teaching process and apply them in practice
- ◆ Describe the different domains of learning
- ◆ Discuss the factors that will affect learning
- ◆ Identify different teaching strategies

◆ Understand some of the approaches that make teaching effective

◆ Select appropriate teaching methods and audiovisual aids to support your teaching.

## WHAT IS LEARNING?

Should you search the literature you will find many definitions of learning; some involve reflection and experience, in addition to the influences of more formal study; almost all involve a relatively permanent change in behaviour.

Certainly in nursing teaching it is the change in behaviour that we wish to bring about if we are to enhance and improve care for patients and clients. For the purpose of this chapter, learning is defined as any event that brings about a relatively permanent change in behaviour, resulting from either experience or practice. Implicit in this is the learned ability to undertake certain procedures or tasks (as you will identify in Activity 3.2) apparently effortlessly and naturally.

It is important to note, however, that dealing solely in definitions is sometimes problematic, as they may imply that teaching and learning are inseparable, whereas in reality it is possible for learning to take place without any noticeable teaching having occurred. However, providing definitions of both teaching and learning that are totally independent of each other is practically impossible.

---

**ACTIVITY 3.1**

Try to identify some instances, either in your personal life or in practice, where you have learned without being actively taught.

There are many examples you may have chosen. In childhood, a great deal of our learning is acquired by experiencing what is happening around us. In practice, many skills – for example supporting bereaved relatives – are learned by observation and participation.

---

For this chapter, it is sufficient for us to accept that if a student is to learn, teaching in some guise is likely to have taken place – and if a teacher is to teach, there must be a student. As a result, throughout this chapter the words 'teaching' and 'learning' will often be used interchangeably.

---

**ACTIVITY 3.2**

Take a few moments to think of the tasks and procedures you are able to do at work which have become 'second nature'. Now, think of everything you did on your last shift at work when you felt you were on 'automatic pilot'.

You will undoubtedly have identified numerous things that you do without being consciously aware of your actions – for example, admitting a patient to the ward or preparing someone for theatre. How we learn to undertake tasks, carry out procedures and deal with particular situations in this way is explained in part by different models of learning.

# Models and theories of learning

Educational psychologists and educationalists have over the years developed models of learning, and a very brief overview follows here. There are many excellent publications and websites available should you wish to explore this area further; see Further Reading at the end of the chapter.

### BEHAVIOURIST

These theories are based on what is termed stimulus and response. This means that the student responds largely to a stimulus, that is, information provided by the teacher, rather than to any other forces. This implies that the student is quite passive in the learning process, and learning is largely dependent on input from others. The emphasis is on 'conditioning' the student to respond in a given way to given situations.

- **Classical conditioning**  Classical conditioning was first described by Pavlov (cited in Curzon 1997), who observed that dogs normally salivated at the sight of food. This he termed an unconditioned response, as it was inherent in the dog without any training being required. Pavlov then sounded a bell before the dog received its food, and discovered it was possible to train the dog to salivate to the ringing of the bell rather than to the production of food, a conditioned response.

- **Operant conditioning**  This theory is also based on stimulus and response, but relies on a system of effective training by using rewards. The psychologist Skinner (1968) discovered that it was possible for pigeons to learn how to operate a lever to deliver their food; the food was both their reward and the factor that reinforced their learning of how to use the lever. He used a 'schedule of re-enforcements' which had to be applied consistently.

You may ask how such a theory can possibly help you, as a practitioner involved in teaching. This is not necessarily a wrong assumption. It is largely supported by Curzon (1997, p. 39), who states that Skinner's 'generalisations concerning human behaviour have been attacked as reflecting the study of animals which are totally unlike human beings. The shaped behaviour of a pigeon taught to dance has been held to be irrelevant to an explanation of the complex activities which form human behaviour'.

Supporters of classical conditioning reason that, although it acknowledges the need for refinement, Pavlov's work can be used to shape the intellectual development of students. This view, much simplified, is based on the fact that he demonstrated that learning is dependent on interaction with the contextual circumstances. For example, students may learn the type of behaviour expected of them in the classroom situation just by being there.

### COGNITIVE OR HUMANISTIC

These theories are more student-centred and are, as a result, much easier to apply in nursing. Cognition means the act of knowing (*Concise Oxford Dictionary* 1999), and involves students' own thinking and perception. The approach centres on the work of Rogers (1983). Rogers includes in the act of knowing the feelings of the student, and the need to recognise his or her individuality – the humanistic approach.

### CONSTRUCTIVIST

This is an extension of the cognitive/humanistic theories of learning. Importance is placed on self-awareness, and the individual's understanding of the processes involved in his or her own learning.

The different views of learning theorists are clearly discussed by Kiger (1995, p. 72), who also, in diagrammatic form, neatly categorises the types of theory we need to consider.

## Domains of learning

Bloom (1972) has identified three areas, or domains, in which learning takes place and which provide a useful framework for the practitioner involved in teaching. These are:

- The **cognitive** domain, concerned with the acquisition of knowledge
- The **psychomotor** domain, relating to the development of skills
- The **affective** domain, involving attitude formation.

The cognitive domain is about how we acquire information, and what we need to know, as opposed to what we need to do. For example, this could be the effects of compression bandaging on a limb, or how insulin works.

The psychomotor domain involves the act of doing, or skills acquisition. This could be learning how to give an intramuscular injection, or how to record an electrocardiogram.

The affective domain relates to the development of beliefs, values and attitudes. An example of this is the acceptance of a patient's right to refuse consent to, or comply with, specific treatment.

The following scenario will help in your understanding of the three domains.

Sister Bell is teaching compression bandaging to a group of students. First, she provides the students with knowledge of the circulatory system and how to identify a venous leg ulcer. This is learning in the cognitive domain.

Next, Sister Bell teaches them how to apply compression bandaging. This lies in the psychomotor domain. Finally, she discusses with the students the patient's attitude to wearing compression bandaging and the need to ensure that it is accepted by the patient if treatment is to be effective. This is learning in the affective domain.

The domains described, known as Bloom's taxonomy, may, according to Curzon, 'assist the teacher in asking the fundamental questions: in what ways should my students have changed as the result of my teaching, and what evidence for the change will I accept?' (Curzon 1997, p. 107).

---

**ACTIVITY 3.3**

Identify a piece of teaching that you have recently undertaken. In which of the domains did learning take place?

It is essential to consider all three domains in our teaching, even though we may not always use them all.

It is unlikely that any single theory or model will account for all aspects of learning that take place, but it would appear that the cognitive theories previously outlined can help students to acquire problem-solving skills that they will require in their future roles. The stimulus–response or conditioning theories, with their emphasis on re-enforcement, point to the importance of immediate feedback in the learning situation.

---

However useful models and theories identifying how we learn may be, there are numerous other factors that are key to effective learning. In particular, we need to consider what issues are important for the adult learner, and how individual differences will affect the learning that takes place.

## Sociological factors affecting learning

The most relevant sociological factors that may influence the learning process are those of language, social class and culture. These are not new to the body of knowledge about how people learn. As far back as 1962, Bernstein identified what he terms a 'restricted language code', which is closely linked to child-rearing practices and education. He argues that people from a working-class background use a limited vocabulary compared with the middle and upper classes, who have a much more elaborate language code. This ultimately affects the way in which people think and make sense of the world around them. If this view is accepted, it would obviously have a bearing on the learning process, as teachers and students would not necessarily be 'speaking the same language'.

Another important aspect of language is that of meaning. This is neatly summed up in the phrase 'I know you think you heard what I said, but what I said is not what I meant!' Put another way, sometimes the words we use may have a different meaning for the person with whom we are communicating. The words of the hospital 'spokesperson' provides us with a perfect example of this: the patient's condition is usually described as 'comfortable' even if the patient is suffering from multiple fractures.

Culture, in its broadest terms, relates to the shared beliefs, values and understanding that are subscribed to by identifying with a particular group. Any student group will link into a culture or subculture of one type or another. For example, patients or clients as a group tend to identify with one another in terms of common problems, and we encourage this by introducing them to self-help groups. The teacher needs to understand the accepted values, attitudes and behaviours of the culture or subculture in order to establish a rapport with the student. Mead (1934) states that we all start off by learning roles from our parents and then complete our socialisation by internalising – that is, accepting as our own – the norms and values of other membership groups, at both the cultural and the subcultural levels. We also tend to become labelled by others according to the cultures and subcultures in which we find ourselves.

The cultural influences brought to bear on students are of enormous consequence, as they may be of far greater importance to the student than those imparted by the teacher. For example, their relationship to their peer group is very important to adolescents, and they would often rather please their peers than their family or teachers. As a result, much of what the teacher tries to achieve will be of no consequence if it is not accepted by the peer group.

For example, if you were teaching health promotion to a group of students, you would need to estimate the influence of their peer group. If your session was on the effects of smoking, it would be easier to demonstrate the ill-effects to a group whose peer group did not smoke and whose original socialisation to non-smoking behaviour was because their parents did not smoke. It would obviously be harder to convince a group of the ill-effects of smoking if their parents had always smoked and members of their peer group also smoked. Teachers must therefore be aware that culture can have a great bearing on the effectiveness of learning.

More recently, Nicklin and Kenworthy (2000) raise the important issue that people from lower social classes generally do less well than their middle-class friends in tests and examinations.

## THE ADULT LEARNER

Traditionally, both pre-registration courses and courses in continuing professional development have been clearly structured, in terms of both content and teaching strategies. Changes in thinking about learning styles and the development of new ways of learning – for example open and distance learning – have led to different approaches being used.

In addition, the increase in project or self-directed work now undertaken by students in secondary education has led to their having different expectations about how they should be taught.

---

**ACTIVITY 3.4**   Think about a course or programme of study you have recently undertaken. Did you feel that the teaching style treated you as a child? What happened to make you feel this way?

For example, the teaching style might not have been adult-centred. It could have been formal, with lots of 'chalk and talk', where the teacher decided what was to be learned. Sessions were kept strictly to time, with little or no discussion and no acknowledgement of individual learning styles within the group.

By contrast, an adult-centred session would be flexible. Recognising the needs of the individual, it would take account of different learning styles and put the student more in control of his or her learning. There would be a large element of discussion, with a degree of negotiation and an element of choice.

---

One of the biggest difficulties when other people are in control of our learning is that we cannot then own it. As a result, we see other people as being responsible for it. Ownership of learning is fundamental to the principles of lifelong learning, which are discussed in Chapter 2.

It is important that, as a practitioner, you are aware of your role in enabling and supporting students to take responsibility for their own learning.

## Androgogy and pedagogy

'The successful teacher is no longer on a height, pumping knowledge at high pressure into passive receptacles ... he is a senior student anxious to help his juniors' (Sir William Osler, 1849–1919).

**ACTIVITY 3.5**

Apart from the fact that the above quotation is less gender friendly than we would expect today, it is difficult to imagine that this was written so long ago. Reflect on what this statement means to you. How far do you agree with it?

Two key issues emerge from this statement. First, effective teaching requires more than just telling someone else what you think they ought to know. Second, the implication is that teaching is helping someone else to learn.

Probably the most straightforward definition of androgogy is provided by Knowles (1984), who defines it as 'the art and science of helping adults to learn'. This is contrasted with pedagogy, which means 'the art and science of teaching children'. Knowles argues that there are fundamental differences in these two approaches that will ultimately affect how students learn.

Androgogy implies that:

- Learning occurs as a result of the student's own effort
- The teacher and students treat each other as equals in the teaching and learning process
- The teaching methods selected are student-centred
- The students accept responsibility for their own learning.

Pedagogy implies that:

- Learning occurs as a result of the input of others
- The student–teacher partnership is unequal – students look up to the teacher
- Teaching methods are teacher-led
- The teacher accepts responsibility for the student's learning.

This idea is further developed by Quinn (2000), who states that teaching can be divided into two broad categories: traditional and progressive. Traditional teaching is characterised by its teacher-centredness, with the student assuming a passive role. The progressive approach is much more student-orientated, with the student playing an active role.

**ACTIVITY 3.6**

From the above, it is clear that an androgogical approach to teaching is different because it involves students being treated as adults. Think of your own experiences as a student. What led you to believe you were being treated as an adult, as opposed to the teacher having responsibility for your learning?

You will probably have identified some of the following:

- There was mutual respect between you and the teacher
- Your teacher was approachable
- He or she showed a willingness to discuss rather than dictate
- The teacher accepted you as a person
- The teacher accepted your personal values.

Rogers (1983) states that effective teaching refers to a set of features that may characterise a number of different processes:

- It must involve learning and possibly teaching
- The content of what is taught must be thought valuable
- The teaching method used must be considered morally acceptable to both the teacher and student.

Rogers also provides us with a very useful framework for practitioners who are involved in teaching in practice:

- **The importance of establishing a climate of trust**   From our own experience we can recognise our need to be accepted as a person, secure in the knowledge that we are valued.

- **Being aware of the individual learning needs of the student**   This involves being aware of the student's current knowledge, for example the stage of training reached and his or her competence in undertaking certain procedures.

- **The importance of student motivation to the learning process**

- **Exposure to a wide range of experiences**

- **Acting as a resource**   This means acting as a 'signpost' in order to direct students to the information they may require. For example, you may need to refer to work that is undertaken in another department, or to highlight available literature.

There are many opportunities in your day-to-day work that can be used as a vehicle to enable your students to learn. Information that is shared and discussed provides an excellent learning opportunity for the student. For the same reason, ward rounds can be of great value. Taking part in a ward round has the added benefit of observing multidisciplinary approaches to care, and makes the student feel part of the team. Involving students in case or care conferences also reinforces the importance of collaboration and cooperation with other organisations and agencies in the provision of patient/client care.

Although we all try to get on with our colleagues, we clearly prefer being with some people rather than others, usually because their personalities are compatible with our own. However, it is likely that at some stage in our careers, and despite great effort on both sides, a personality clash will be unavoidable. In such a case it is better to discuss it openly with all the parties involved so that the issue can be addressed in the best interests of all.

- **Sharing the student's thoughts and feelings**    This involves all aspects of 'being there' for the student, and sharing feelings in relation to events in the practice situation. It also means making the student feel wanted as a learner. It is important for us, as practitioners, to remember that for every nurse who has been aware of supervising a disinterested student there is a student who feels that he or she has had a disinterested facilitator or mentor.

- **Using conflict and tensions as a learning experience**    This means talking through with the student distressing or disturbing experiences that he or she may have encountered. For example, decisions taken regarding patient resuscitation can be extremely upsetting when first encountered by students.

- **Accepting one's own strengths and weaknesses**    Implicit in this is the need for you, as a facilitator, to accept your own limitations, safe in the knowledge that you cannot know everything there is to know about your area of practice, or be all things to all people. Accepting your own strengths and weaknesses requires you to look objectively at yourself and try to improve on some aspects of your role, while at the same time acknowledging that at which you are proficient.

## Superficial versus deep learning

After reading this section you should be able to understand your own approach to learning more clearly. It is a useful framework to remind you to encourage your students to become deep as opposed to superficial learners.

Superficial learning is exactly what it implies – it is scraping the surface of the material being studied, without carrying out any deep processing of the material itself.

Students who do this tend to:

- Concentrate on assessment requirements (it is easy for an experienced teacher to spot this)

- Accept information and ideas passively
- Memorise facts and procedures as a matter of routine
- Ignore any patterns or guiding principles
- Fail to reflect on any underlying strategy or purpose.

Students who adopt a deep approach to learning try to turn other people's ideas into their own personalised structure of knowledge. Such students tend to:

- Try to make sense of content and issues themselves
- Be critical of the content
- Apply what is being learned to their previous knowledge and experience
- Use organising principles to integrate their ideas
- Find evidence to underpin conclusions
- Explore the logic of arguments.

Students who adopt a strategic approach to learning in this way set out with a plan of action to obtain the highest grades possible. Generally, they:

- Maintain a balanced approach to study
- Locate the right materials with which to do the work
- Are fully aware of what is required in terms of assessment criteria
- Are alert to the different roles in the student–teacher relationship.

If students are to reach their potential throughout their lifelong learning, then it is crucial to the process that they become deep learners.

## THE IMPORTANCE OF INDIVIDUAL DIFFERENCES

Ewan and White (1996) highlight the importance of getting to know students' individual characteristics and needs, if learning is to be effective. This is largely a result of the individual's own learning style, sometimes referred to as their cognitive style.

Research undertaken by psychologists has identified basic differences in our preferred way of learning (Hudson 1968, Pask 1976). Put simply, there are many different ways in which we approach and process information. For example, some students find the use of diagrams helpful when learning, whereas others prefer to rely solely on the written word.

| TABLE 3.1 | *Four categories of learning style* | | | |
| --- | --- | --- | --- | --- |
| | **Activists** | **Reflectors** | **Theorists** | **Pragmatists** |
| | Like novelty<br>Energetic<br>Easily bored<br>Open-minded<br>Enjoy working<br>  alongside others<br>Live for the present | Like time to think<br>Thorough<br>Avoid reaching<br>  speedy conclusions<br>Are observers as<br>  opposed to leaders | Analyse situations<br>Systematic<br>Have the ability to<br>  reason<br>Need to know logic<br>  behind actions and<br>  observations | Learning dictated by<br>  practical consequences,<br>  rather than theory<br>Receptive to new ideas<br>Like things to happen<br>  quickly |

Honey and Mumford (cited in Stengelhofen 1996, pp. 54–55) identify four distinct learning styles that are useful in helping us to understand individual learning needs. They state that the students can be categorised into activists, pragmatists, theorists or reflectors (Table 3.1).

| ACTIVITY 3.7 | What characteristics do you think individuals would possess in each of the four categories?<br><br>  The names that have been given to the four categories provide us with a very good indication of the preferred learning style of the individual. |
| --- | --- |

| ACTIVITY 3.8 | Think where your own learning style, or those of your students, may lie in relation to the four categories identified.<br><br>  Although the above list provides only a short description, it is clear that the teaching method we use could affect whether the student will learn new information. For example, a student who has an activist learning style may have difficulty learning from a lecture in which there is no student interaction. A reflector may find learning from role-play problematic, as that would depend on an immediate response from the student. Varying your teaching methods will undoubtedly appeal to your students' different learning styles. |
| --- | --- |

## MOTIVATION

It is impossible to think about how we learn without thinking about why we want to do it! To say that a person must want to learn in order for learning to take place seems self-evident, but there are many factors (within both the teaching and the learning process) that will contribute to the student's wish to learn. Motivation, according to Sargent (1990, p. 4) 'is about what makes people tick'. For example, what makes a student who has completed a

diploma course move on to a degree? Or an overworked ward manager stay on the ward after his or her span of duty has finished?

Motivation can be described as either intrinsic or extrinsic to the individual. Intrinsic motivation relates to the personal factors that make us want to learn. The theorist Maslow (1987) provides a good example of intrinsic motivation. He identifies five levels of need that must be met for a person to reach his or her fullest potential:

1. **Physiological**   When applied to student learning, this means that if the student environment is, for example, over or underheated, or noisy – or if the student is tired – learning is unlikely to take place, or may be limited.

2. **Safety**   Students need to feel safe from danger at every level. For example, students may feel 'unsafe' in an environment where they do not know other students, or do not have confidence in the teacher.

3. **Social**   This involves the 'need to be needed' (or valued) in both our home and our working life, for example to be accepted by our colleagues.

4. **Self-esteem**   When applied to student learning, self-esteem means the need for mutual respect between the individual student, the students as a group, and the teacher.

5. **Self-actualisation**   Maslow claims that it is only when these individual needs have been met that the student is able to reach their full potential and have the opportunity to 'become everything one is capable of becoming' (Sargent 1990, p. 5).

There are, however, other intrinsic factors that will influence learning – for example, your personal feelings regarding your relationship with other students and teachers.

Extrinsic motivation is that which occurs outside the student, and over which he or she may have no control. It is important to note here that the two types of motivation are rarely exclusive of each other. For example, the way in which students are welcomed on to the ward or clinic will undoubtedly affect how they feel – no one likes to feel unwelcome!

| ACTIVITY 3.9 | Think of a course of study you have recently undertaken. Try to identify the factors that made you want to learn. Were these intrinsic, extrinsic, or a mixture of both? |
| --- | --- |

If the course of study you identified was in nursing, it is likely that you identified some of the extrinsic factors of motivation – for example the need to pass examinations in order to practice in a particular role or specialism. Indeed, your salary or promotion may depend on it.

Ewan and White (1996) argue that these two aspects are by no means exclusive of each other, as students of nursing normally enter education with a high degree of intrinsic motivation. This can then be overtaken by extrinsic factors, particularly the need to pass examinations. They go on to say that this is the reason why, in teaching, some students 'are only interested in what they will be asked in the exams' (p. 45).

# THE VALUE OF REFLECTIVE PRACTICE TO THE TEACHING AND LEARNING PROCESS

You will already have identified from your experiences of continuing professional development the value of reflective practice both to the teacher and to the whole of the learning process. The principles of this are particularly relevant to this chapter, both in terms of enhancing the learning experience for the student and in helping you, as a practitioner and a teacher, to develop your teaching skills.

Reflection is about analysing a situation in order to decide on the best way forward and to learn from it. Boud et al. (1985) identify a preparatory phase in the reflective process in which the student consciously anticipates the experience. It is argued that this is an essential part of learning and that its value should not be overlooked. In view of this, reflection is concerned with looking forward to experiences as well as learning from what has passed.

There are four key points that are crucial to becoming proficient in the process of reflective practice:

1. The need for conscious and voluntary effort.

2. Its usefulness as a tool in helping you to explore the links between what you are told and your observations in practice.

3. The importance of journal writing in assisting the reflective process.

4. The need to work through initial difficulties in journal writing as these diminish with persistence and practice.

Wallace (1999) argues that most nurses in the past had already adopted reflective practice, although it may not have been known under that particular title.

# THE IMPORTANCE OF JOURNAL, LOG OR DIARY WRITING TO LEARNING

This has become a popular method of learning, particularly when the learning is self-directed. Journals provide a very useful tool from which to explore beliefs and values in terms of your own experiences. They can also provide a very powerful teaching tool when used as the basis for group discussion or in one-to-one tutorials. This aspect will be discussed in greater depth later in this chapter.

The main aim of a journal is to help you or your student to develop skills of reflection, evaluation and decision-making. However, probably the most important aspect for you, as a practitioner, is its place in helping to forge the links between theory and practice.

## How to write a journal

One of the key aspects that must be stressed in relation to personal journals is that of confidentiality. This is implicit in the Nursing and Midwifery Council Code of professional conduct (NMC) 2002. No material written in the journal should make it possible to identify any patient or client by either name or inference.

Dewing (1990) identifies some useful ground rules if personal journals are to form the basis of group discussion:

1. The journal is the property of the nurse who writes it.

2. Writers are free to reveal as much or as little of the content of their journal as they wish.

3. Shared information is not to be revealed to others without consent.

4. Comments on other nurses' reflections must be positive and supportive.

5. Nurses commenting on each others' reflections must work together as a peer group.

With the increased emphasis on reflective practice as a valuable contributor to the teaching process, it is natural to assume that it is a relatively new concept. However, probably the most straightforward definition of a journal as a reflective tool was provided by Baldwin (1977, p. 10), who differentiated between a journal and a diary by describing a diary as a record of observations and experiences, and a journal as a 'tool for recording the process of our lives'.

Generally speaking, diaries are much more superficial and are used for recording day-to-day events. Journals may not only contain experiences and activities, but also incorporate the writer's reflections and the impact that these have on his or her life. Prognoff (1975) argues that maintaining a journal provides continuity for the student by enabling her to reflect on specific events and periods, record them, and then carry out a dialogue, linking past and present events and reactions to them. Journals can be very helpful during times of change brought about by circumstances external to the writer. Reviewing how one handled previous changes may offer strategies for how to handle the present situation.

Writing thoughts and feelings may be cathartic in itself. Prognoff (1975) found that reading aloud made a stronger impact on the reader than did silent reading. Journals also have the advantage of allowing the writer to return to past entries and reread them in order to gain some insight into the present.

## Recording your journal

How you actually record is a matter of personal choice. Looseleaf notebooks provide much greater flexibility as pages can be added and removed when required. Whatever its format, the journal should be used solely for the purpose of recording your journal entries; that is, it should not be used to jot down telephone messages or patient notes, for example. Some practical tips on keeping a journal are outlined in Box 3.1.

The implementation of the United Kingdom Central Council's (UKCC) post-registration education and practice (PREP 1994) requirements has led to an increase in the use of reflective diaries as a means of demonstrating how learning has influenced patient/client care. This has, in turn, led to concern regarding who should have access to the information contained within

---

**BOX 3.1**

- Remember that the main aim of the journal is your own development
- It is not as much work as it appears. The more you use it the easier it becomes
- Be brief. Only write as much as is necessary to get your point across, but avoid just making lists
- Try to focus on the now of your life or the very recent past, or past few days
- Make at least one positive statement about yourself, your strengths and or your abilities in each entry
- Review your entry every month and rewrite all the positive comments you have made about yourself during that time
- Your journal is private to you so you can be totally honest with yourself
- Do not analyse too much by rereading your entries
- Take great care to ensure that the patient/client is not identifiable. The journal is private to you, but we are all human and things get mislaid.

such diaries. For example, in the unlikely event of the patient or client discussed in the journal or diary being the focus of court proceedings, could the contents be used as evidence? To date, there are no known instances of this occurring so it is difficult to forecast its possibility. However, while there is even the slightest possibility that portfolio entries could be relevant in litigation, it is crucial that you make it impossible to recognise any patient or client in your journal. Taking time to think how you are going to achieve this is an integral part of maintaining your journal or diary. In addition, a useful tip at the end of each entry is to ask yourself the fundamental question: 'Would anyone be able to identify the patient or client from what I have written?' If they could, the entry must be reworded.

An excellent introduction to reflective journals is provided by Ghaye (1996).

## LINKING THEORY WITH PRACTICE: THE ROLE OF THE PRACTITIONER

As a practitioner you are likely to be aware of the term 'theory–practice gap'. The fundamental mistake we make is that we see it as a new problem brought about by changes in both the education and the practice of nursing. However, it is not a new concept, and as long as 50 years ago the need for theory and practice to be integrated was highlighted.

In addition, there are many different perceptions of what has become termed the theory–practice gap, making the issue extremely complex (Welsh and Swan 2002). Before we look at your role in bridging it, it is essential to identify what you, as a practitioner, perceive to be a theory–practice gap.

| ACTIVITY 3.10 | Think about your current role. Do you believe there to be a gap in the application of practice to theory? If so, why do you think this is? |
|---|---|

The aspects you have identified will depend on your current role and will probably include one or more of the following:

- Theory being purely 'academic', for example, where it is not used in practice
- Nursing students not being able to transfer what they have learned in the classroom to the practical situation
- A lack of contact with the teachers providing the theory
- A lack of information from the institution providing the theory.

Although the reasons for the theory–practice gap are diverse, there are many ways in which you, as a practitioner, can close it. These are by gaining an understanding of the curriculum and processes in operation where these affect you in your work (see the section on the curriculum, below).

You have probably included in your answer aspects such as having an understanding of what students are being taught in theory, your own attitudes and beliefs, the time available, levels of motivation etc. From this, it is clear that journal writing is only one way in which we can build links between theory and practice.

# TEACHING STRATEGIES

Now that we have explored the issues that may have a strong influence on how students learn and what may help their learning, we can examine some of the strategies we can adopt in order to ensure our teaching is effective.

Even the most confident and competent of teachers will admit to a degree of nervousness when asked to undertake a presentation for the first time, but with the right approach and preparation this can become a very enjoyable part of the practitioner's role. The purpose of this part of the chapter is, therefore, to provide you with the 'how to' of teaching by giving you a framework within which to make your teaching effective. It will identify strategies that you can employ in order to maximise your students' learning and enable you to plan your teaching appropriately.

## Building the framework: why we need a teaching strategy

A strategy, in its simplest form, is concerned with forward planning. The *Concise Oxford Dictionary* (1999) describes it as 'the art of war; especially the part of it concerned with the conduct of campaigns'. This may appear to be a rather extreme definition, but those of you who have had the experience of teaching a group of over 250 pre-registration diploma students are unlikely to deny the need to be organised. What is also apparent is that, as individuals, we all have different concerns and worries regarding our teaching and how it is received.

Jolly (1997) suggests that the transition from being a student teacher to being a qualified teacher in the classroom situation is problematic, particularly regarding integration. This is largely because the teacher has not yet developed a sense of belonging in relation to the educational establishment concerned. Clifford (1995) also cites conflicts and challenges for nurse teachers as they attempt to meet the diverse aspects of their role. It could be argued that this is equally applicable to practitioners who are asked to teach in similar circumstances. As a practitioner and as a teacher, then, the starting point is one of survival.

## Teaching a skill

Teaching skills are probably an important aspect of the role of practitioners, either in teaching patients/clients to undertake a particular procedure for themselves or teaching student nurses skills, such as the safe moving and handling of patients.

As experienced practitioners, many of the skills that you undertake in your daily work, for example the positioning of your feet prior to moving a patient, are largely carried out subconsciously. It is likely that, because of the amount of practice you have had at performing the procedure, it has become instinctive.

We have learned from earlier chapters that learning is enhanced if the material is provided in a logical sequence. This is particularly relevant when teaching a skill, as the action can be broken down into a series of stages or steps. Skills teaching involves learning in both the cognitive and the motor domains.

---

**ACTIVITY 3.11**

Imagine that you have a new student nurse on your ward and you want to teach her how to administer drugs safely from the trolley. Write down the steps you would need to go through in order to complete the task.

You will want to check the following items, although their order may change depending on your individual preference:

- The drug bottle label against the patient's drug administration record
- The dosage of the drug
- The time the drug is to be given
- That it is being given to the correct patient by asking him or her
- The name on the patient's armband to confirm this
- That the patient does not have any allergies to the drug about to be given.

---

If skills can be broken down as a series of steps they are much more easily understood, although there are other factors for us to consider, for example the level of motivation of the student and how the subject is presented by the teacher.

## Preparing your teaching

One of the greatest difficulties for most practitioners faced with teaching for the first time is where to start. As identified earlier in the chapter, it is clear that the teaching method you select may affect the way in which students learn, so an assessment of your student or student group is essential.

**ACTIVITY 3.12**  Think about the types of experience that are available in your area of work and how you could ensure that the students have access to these.

Your answer will undoubtedly reflect your personal learning style. There is, however, a sequence of events that can be applied regardless of the method selected. There is an old adage that is well known to teachers:

Tell 'em what you're going to tell 'em.
Then tell 'em.
Then tell 'em what you've just told 'em!

This principle can be applied to other situations. Next time you have the opportunity to view one of the old Hollywood slapstick comedies with the 'custard pie in the face' routine, watch carefully the sequence of events:

1. The 'deliverer' of the custard pie indicates what is going to happen, i.e. he is going to let the 'receiver' have it in the face! (Tell 'em what you're going to tell 'em.)

2. The 'deliverer' delivers said custard pie to the 'recipient'. (Then tell 'em.)

3. The 'deliverer' holds empty plate, indicates the content on 'receiver's' face and laughs. (Tell 'em what you've just told 'em!)

The sequence of events when planning teaching is therefore:

● The introduction

● The progression of the subject material

● The conclusion.

The introduction includes 'setting the scene' for the session, finding out what the students already know, and telling them why they need to learn the knowledge and the method by which they are to learn it. Equally as important, regardless of the teaching method you choose, is the way in which you communicate with your students.

## Communication skills

As we saw earlier in this chapter, recent years have seen dramatic changes in the way we are taught, moving from a pedagogical to an androgogical approach. Fundamental to this approach is the way in which we communicate our teaching material. The following are some general rules to follow, both in preparation and during your teaching:

- Ask open as opposed to closed questions, for example:
  - What do you understand by that?
  - How would you do this?
  - What other view might you consider?

- Show an understanding of other people's feelings. You may be nervous teaching, but the student may also be afraid to speak.

- Listen carefully to what a student has to say.

- Silence is possibly one of the most difficult situations to deal with when teaching, and 20 seconds' silence when you have posed a question really does seem like a lifetime. This makes you vulnerable to answering your own questions rather than waiting for the student's response.

---

**ACTIVITY 3.13**

Position yourself as if you were speaking at the front of the class and ask a question (it doesn't matter what). Now wait 20 seconds. You will soon learn how long this can feel.

- Give students alternatives. There is often more than one way of achieving the same goal.
- Make sure that your facts are correct.
- Do not be afraid of saying that you do not have an answer. Teachers never could, nor should they, know everything.
- Admit it openly if you get something wrong.

---

## The use of humour in teaching

Parkin (1989) argues that, when used properly, humour is one of the most important qualities of a good teacher. There is only one major rule regarding the use of humour in your teaching: it should be appropriate and linked closely with the content of your teaching.

Having looked at some of the general issues, the following is a basic, but nonetheless useful, framework to use that will help you to feel more confident. It is often termed the 'what, why, when, where and how of teaching'.

## The what of teaching

This aspect is not always quite as straightforward as it sounds, and many practitioners make the mistake of overlooking it. For example, you may be asked to deliver a teaching session on the moving and handling of patients, but what aspects of moving and handling are you required to teach? In reality, this can encompass legislation, aids to assist moving and handling, patient safety, nurse safety and employer policy. The possibilities are almost endless. This lesson was brought home to me very early in my teaching career when I was asked to deliver 10 hours' teaching on the learning environment!

Using the following as a guide will assist you in deciding exactly what you want the students to learn:

- First, seek a clear answer to the fundamental question of what part of the subject you are being asked to teach. This will not only reduce your stress levels, but also enable you to focus your teaching and ensure that you are not repeating content that has already been taught.

- Having identified the subject matter (you may sometimes have to be quite persistent about this), you are then in a position to develop the aim and specific objectives for the session (see below). Although it is acknowledged that the formulation of objectives may not always be the best way to plan your teaching, it does enable you, if you are new to teaching, to be much more focused.

## The importance of evidence-based practice

Evidence-based practice has been described as the bridge between research and practice (Curzio 1997). As something we carry out, evidence-based practice is 'about finding, appraising and applying scientific evidence to the treatment and management of healthcare' (Hamer and Collinson 1999, p. 6).

It is therefore incumbent on the teacher to ensure that her teaching materials are from the same evidence-base. This can be achieved by always ensuring that you research your subject fully, and by providing the students with the evidence to support your statements and views.

One of the key purposes of evidence-based practice is to ensure that the patient/client receives up-to-date care based on up to date knowledge. It is, therefore, vital to the learning process that your information is not based on 'history'. The easiest way of ensuring this is by undertaking a literature search on the subject you are intending to teach. Your College of Nursing library will be able to assist you in this. It is important that your search is highly focused on what you want to know. For example, if you entered the words 'nursing process' you would get over 1000 'hits', which is obviously not much help. By asking yourself what exactly it is that you wish to know about the nursing process, you will narrow the subject down drastically and the information you receive will be much more manageable and pertinent.

## The why of teaching

In order for you to gain an understanding of what is required in terms of teaching, it is essential to know why a particular subject is to be taught. For example:

- Is the subject an examinable part of the curriculum?
- If this is the case, what aspects of the subject must the students know?
- Does it link with previously taught subjects?

## The when of teaching

There are five fundamental questions that you may find useful:

1. How much time have you been allocated for the session?
2. Is the time sufficient for what you have been asked to do?
3. How does what you have been asked to teach fit into the module or course? For example, is it a 'standalone' session or one of a series?
4. If others are teaching on the same subject, how can you ensure that there is no overlap or repetition?
5. How will your teaching and the students' learning be evaluated?

## The where of teaching

This may appear self-explanatory, but the changing numbers of student groups and the frequent, limited use of classroom accommodation often lead to various annexed buildings being used. It may be that your teaching is to take place in the practice area. If so, you will need to consider exactly where to carry out the teaching in order to avoid any distractions.

## The how of teaching

Having gained the above information and established your objectives, you are now in a position to decide what is the most appropriate teaching method for the subject material you are to deliver.

# PROVIDING A STRUCTURE FOR TEACHING

## Aims and objectives

The development of aims and objectives as a framework for a planned teaching session is extremely useful. First, they provide a logical sequence for both you and your student, and second, they enable you to check whether your teaching has been effective. Central to the development of aims and objectives is the decision about what exactly the student should learn.

## Identifying what to teach

This is often described as the must, should and could of teaching, and although it is a simple framework it will provide you with some very useful pegs on which to hang your subject material.

**ACTIVITY 3.14**

Think of a subject of which you have a sound knowledge. Here are some examples to help with your choice:

- Accidental hypothermia in older people
- Storing drugs safely
- Planning off-duty rotas
- Care of a patient immediately following surgery.

To take the safe storage of drugs as an example, you may feel that the students must know the following:

- The law relating to drug storage
- Your employer's policy on storage
- The process of recording stored drugs.

What they *should* know – that is, desirable additions to the *must-knows* – are the wider issues involved, for example the ordering and disposal of stored drugs. Finally, what the students *could* know – that is, non-essential but optional knowledge – is the patient's/client's role in storage.

This can provide a useful framework for identifying what is the most important content of your teaching and so should enable you to formulate its aim.

## Identifying your aim for the session

An aim in teaching terms is an overall statement that identifies what the student must be able to do at the end of a given period of instruction or experience.

**ACTIVITY 3.15** With this definition in mind, try to formulate an aim for the subject that you identified in Activity 3.14.

There are two key aspects to remember when identifying your aim: first, it is a general statement of what is to be achieved; and second, it should state why it is worth achieving.

To use the example of accidental hypothermia in older people, the aim for the teaching would be something like: 'At the end of the session, students will understand the nature of accidental hypothermia in older people, so that they can deliver skilled nursing care'. You will notice that the aim does not tell you how this will be achieved. This is done in the next step, by formulating educational objectives or what are now often called (intended) learning outcomes.

Generally speaking, objectives or learning outcomes must:

- Be achievable within the period allocated for the teaching

- Be specific in terms of what you want the student to achieve

- Be measurable in terms of their outcome.

Again, to use the risk of accidental hypothermia in older people as an example, the educational objectives could be as follows:

At the end of the session students should be able to:

- Explain the predisposing causes of accidental hypothermia in older people

- Recognise the signs and symptoms of accidental hypothermia in this client group

- Describe the treatment of a patient suffering from accidental hypothermia

- Recognise the factors that make older people more at risk of accidental hypothermia.

As a general rule by which to measure your objectives or learning outcomes, always ask whether they are SMART:

1. Specific

2. Measurable

3. Achievable

4. **R**ealistic

5. **T**ime-limited.

Useful as SMART objectives are in helping you to decide what to teach, they do have certain limitations.

| ACTIVITY 3.16 | Make a list of all the positive and negative aspects of teaching by objectives that you can think of. The positive aspects may include that they: |
|---|---|

Make a list of all the positive and negative aspects of teaching by objectives that you can think of. The positive aspects may include that they:

- Provide your teaching with a clear and logical structure
- Enable the teacher to control the timing
- Make it easier to ascertain what the student has learned
- Provide a clear record of what has been taught
- Enable students to direct their own study.

The negative aspects may include that they:

- Are time-consuming to prepare (although this improves with practice)
- Tend to be inflexible
- Limit the content of the session and, as a result, what the student will learn.

On balance, if you are new to teaching, using objectives when preparing to teach is invaluable.

There is a wealth of information available to assist you in formulating your educational objectives. You may find the text by Nicklin and Kenworthy (2000) particularly useful.

## FORMAL AND INFORMAL TEACHING

Teaching is often described as being either formal or informal. Formal refers to the type of teaching that is preplanned, often with a clear aim and objectives. Informal teaching refers to the spontaneous type of teaching that occurs when a situation presents itself.

Formal learning may include areas such as the safe moving and handling of patients, or the care of essential equipment. Informal teaching could include the changing of intravenous fluids, which the student can observe at the bedside. Both types of teaching have advantages and disadvantages.

The major advantages of using a formal method are that usually both the student and teacher know exactly what the session aims to achieve. Further, the formal method enables the student to undertake his or her own preparation – for example by selecting some background reading. The major advantages of using an informal method are that it is meaningful for the student, and helps to ensure that the knowledge he or she is gaining is up-to-date. This is often regarded as a form of action learning.

# DECIDING WHAT TO TEACH

Clearly, in nurse education programmes decisions have to be taken about what the students should learn. Abbatt and McMahon (1993, p. 17) describe this succinctly:

> ...if there is a course for orthopaedic surgeons, it should be totally different from a course for health inspectors. Health inspectors do not need to be able to replace hip joints, and orthopaedic surgeons do not need to control the breeding sites of mosquitoes.

In the same way, nurse education programmes need to be relevant to the area of work that students will be expected to undertake on completion of the course. This is achieved by curriculum planning, and the selection of an appropriate curriculum model with which to design the course.

Many of you reading this chapter will be familiar with using nursing models to plan and prioritise care. In the same way, formalised programmes of nurse education are based on curriculum models. A curriculum model, as defined by Burrel (1988), is the organised setting out of the key elements of what should be learned, either using the written word or in diagrammatic form.

This section will provide you with a brief introduction to curriculum models. For those who require a more in-depth knowledge, an excellent outline of curriculum planning and curriculum design is given by Quinn (2000).

The **product model** of curriculum design is based on the 'end result' of education (usually an award or qualification) and the need to meet specific objectives. Learning is seen as a change in observable behaviour, and is measured against the students' achievement of the objectives.

The **process model** of curriculum design depicts learning as intrinsically beneficial, rather than in terms of outcomes. Students are allowed to develop at their own pace; there are no set objectives, and as a result what is learned may be unpredictable.

The use of a product model in some aspects of nurse teaching can be extremely useful, especially when the completion of an end product of learning is required – for example the teaching of fire evacuation procedures to a new student on the ward.

The process model is much more focused on the development of understanding, and so requires a more active role from students. It allows them to develop the skills they need at their own pace. In this model the teacher acts as a facilitator, supporting rather than telling the student what to do. There are no set outcomes to achieve by a given time – for example, the student learns over time how to prioritise care.

As a practitioner, facilitator or teacher, it is important that you are familiar with the curriculum design of the courses with which you are involved. The following is a useful list of questions to ask when talking about this with a relevant lecturer–practitioner:

- What is the philosophy on which the curriculum is based?
- Which curriculum model has been chosen, and why?
- How do the different parts fit together to provide an overall package for the students? For example, how are the students able to relate theory to practice and vice versa?
- How is progression demonstrated throughout the curriculum?
- Does the curriculum allow for differences in learning style?
- Does the curriculum allow for different teaching methods?
- How is the curriculum assessed?
- Does the model allow the student to take responsibility for his or her own learning?

# DIFFERENT APPROACHES TO TEACHING

As stated earlier, the terms teaching and learning are often used interchangeably. It is therefore appropriate to explore some additional conditions that are helpful to our understanding of the teaching process.

## Creating a good environment for teaching

The environment is wherever students are taught. However, it is well recognised from student feedback that the clinical situation is a particularly rich environment for teaching and learning, in that students' motivation to learn is high during their practical experience (see below). This would seem to confirm that the place where students are most likely to be receptive to teaching and learning is the practice setting. This, in turn, makes it important that practitioners involved in teaching know how to create an environment conducive to learning.

**ACTIVITY 3.17**

What key elements do you think are essential in creating a good environment for your students? To what extent do they exist in your own working environment? If they do not, how can you foster them?

You may have identified the need to be:

- Approachable
- Welcoming
- Confident enough in your work to pass information on to others
- Supportive
- Helpful
- Available and contactable
- Knowledgeable.

It is obvious that the more comfortable and safe we feel with the environment, the more likely it is that effective learning will take place.

Some of the aspects you have included in your answer will be developed further below.

## TEACHING METHODS

Having identified what it is that you are going to teach and the environment in which you are going to teach it, you are then in a position to select an appropriate teaching method. There are many different methods that you can use, each of which has its advantages and disadvantages. However, the method selected needs to correspond to the domain of learning in which it is to take place if the learning is to be effective. A lecture is of little value if you wish to change students' attitudes on a given subject – for example, it is highly unlikely that you would change a student's opinion that inequalities in health care were justifiable by just lecturing to him or her.

The method chosen will also depend on the number of students you are going to teach, and there may be occasions when, because of the large number of students involved, the lecture is the only appropriate method. There is a variety of teaching methods that you can use:

- Lectures

- Group discussions

- Seminars

- Role-play

- Learning from critical incidents

- Independent/directed learning
- Experiential learning.

The terms 'lecture' and 'lesson' are frequently used interchangeably, although a lesson tends to imply more student interaction. The lecture largely involves the teacher doing most of the talking, with the students listening. This is an extremely valuable teaching method when you wish to provide the students with particular knowledge – for example the functions of the liver, or the results of certain research.

The lecture is extremely efficient in terms of teacher time as, in so far as accommodation allows, the session can be delivered to large numbers of students at the same time. It is also a very useful way of introducing new topics, which may act as a motivator for the students. Further, the knowledge you provide can be totally up-to-date.

Finally, the lecture provides a useful framework on which to base other sessions. For example, the students may all be given the same information in a lecture, and may then break up into smaller groups to discuss it.

Some of the criticisms levelled at the lecture method are derogatory at best. Auden (cited in Curzon 1997, p. 191), states that 'the lecturer is a person who talks in someone else's sleep'. This might at first glance be a bit off-putting to the new lecturer, but should instil in us the need to make the subject we are going to teach of interest. Some other criticisms of the lecture method are that:

- The students are mainly passive (although the students may see this as a plus!).

- Lectures may not appeal to the student's individual learning style.

- The opportunity to explore the issues raised is limited.

- Finally, it is difficult for the teacher to ascertain whether he or she has been understood.

## Handouts

These are a useful tool that gives students a record of what you have taught during the lecture. They have the added advantage of enabling the student to concentrate on what you are saying, rather than taking notes. Whether or not you use them, however, will depend on the time you have in which to prepare them and the facilities you have available to produce them. There are two basic types: the handout on which you provide all the key points of your lecture, and the 'gapped' handout, which gives the student the main headings and space between each one to enable him or her to complete it during the lecture.

There are five key areas that you should include in a handout:

- The topic being taught
- The aim and objectives (or learning outcomes) of the session
- A statement of the main thrust of the presentation
- A summary of the key points
- An up-to-date list of further reading that students can access if they require more information.

If you were to present a lecture on the effects of smoking on health, a gapped handout would look something like Figure 3.1. The student then completes the handout from the information given during the lecture.

## Delivering a lecture

Beitz (1994) has identified six basic steps that are useful to follow before delivering a lecture:

- Planning
- Writing a detailed outline
- Rehearsing
- Selecting examples
- Knowing the content
- Choosing visual aids.

As Beitz (1994) writes, 'a good oral presentation is an inspiring experience in which learners' minds are broadened, and their interests piqued'. You may wish to add: 'and the teacher survives!'. There is a substantial amount of literature available to support the view that the teacher can learn very useful techniques without too much difficulty (Cooper 1989).

Varying your teaching methods will appeal to students' different learning styles, and even within the lecture you should try to introduce some change of activity – for example the use of audiovisual aids or gapped handouts – and allow time for questions during and after the session.

The next step is writing a detailed outline. There is a fine balance to be drawn here. First, it is tempting to write down all that you know on a particular

FIGURE 3.1    *A gapped handout*

---

### The effects of smoking on health

**Learning outcomes**

At the end of the session, students should be able to:

● Discuss the ways in which smoking affects health

● Describe two of the major health promotion models used to educate

  people to stop smoking

**Questions**

1    What are the effects of smoking on health in the following domains?

● Physical

● Social

● Psychological

● Economic

2    What are the major models used in health promotion?

(i)

(ii)

**Further reading**
Provide a list of relevant material which the students will find useful.

---

subject, and then to read it to the group. This should be avoided at all costs, as it does not allow for student interaction and potentially makes the teaching session both short and boring. Furthermore, it gives the impression that the teacher wants to control the learners, rather than learning alongside them.

The preparation of teaching notes will help you to start planning your teaching session. You will find that the preparation is initially extremely time-consuming, but becomes much quicker with practice. Your teaching plan can also be updated, so it can be used again. As a result, your portfolio of prepared material is gradually built up. Your notes are also a very useful prompt when teaching, to keep you on course.

- Keep your notes reasonably short, but always include the outcomes or objectives for the session and explain their relevance.

- Highlight important points on your plan by using a highlighter pen or red ink. This will ensure you do not omit any information crucial to your teaching.

- Fasten your papers together securely, or ensure that they are adequately numbered (if you are extremely nervous and drop them, you will need to be able to reorder them quickly).

- Make sure that your plan follows a logical sequence, with a clear introduction, middle and end. Use the introduction to outline what you intend to do and its relevance, the middle section to provide the new information, and the summary to 'pull together' the main points. As the old adage runs: 'tell 'em what you're going to tell 'em; tell 'em; and then tell 'em what you've told 'em'.

Now you are ready to rehearse your session. There are unfortunately no shortcuts to this, as timing is crucial if teaching is to be effective. Many of us have, unfortunately, experienced the teaching session that has run way over time, leaving the students tense, irritable and totally switched off. The answer to this potential problem lies in rehearsal, possibly in front of a friend. The confidence that you can gain from doing this is tremendous. First, it enables you to become much more conversant with your subject matter, and second, it ensures that you will not run out of material in the first five minutes.

To illustrate the points you are making, you need to choose some practical examples from your own area of work. For example, if a community nurse is teaching about the safe storage of drugs in the client's home, it becomes much more meaningful to the student if this can be applied to her own experiences, and so helps to bring the teaching to life.

When planning your presentation, it is always worth asking yourself what relevant examples you can use to link theory with practice, but beware of relying too heavily on stories from your own practice unless they are totally pertinent to what you are teaching.

An aspect of teaching you can never ignore is knowing the content. This is probably the only place where no amount of strategic planning will help: you must have an understanding of your subject material and the major concepts involved. Beitz (1994) argues that a willingness to share with the students the learning strategies you have used to assimilate the material may aid their understanding.

It is also useful (and will save you from embarrassment) if you have a reserve of knowledge over and above that which you are going to teach. By doing this, you will not be thrown off course by most questions the group may raise. On the other hand, there is no disgrace in a teacher not knowing the answer to a question, and to say so is far preferable to bluffing your way through. Thankfully, the days when a teacher was expected to know everything are long gone.

# Discussion and tutorial groups

These are best used when there are small groups of students. Between 12 and 15 is ideal, as larger numbers make it difficult to take individual contributions. All of the methods are useful in enabling students to develop their skills in decision-making.

### TUTORIAL GROUPS

These are usually used as a back-up to information already being given by other methods. For example, a tutorial group may look at specific issues raised during a lecture, or may want to discuss the best way in which students can prepare themselves for an important examination. These groups are normally teacher-led, so the teacher needs a good understanding of what is to be discussed to enable the students to reach their conclusions.

Small group discussions are best suited to the following activities:

- Brainstorming
- Snowballing
- Buzz groups
- The presentation of projects or assignments
- Problem-solving.

Brainstorming is a way of collecting ideas from all of the individuals in the group on how to deal with a particular problem. The students state their ideas on a particular issue, and these are then written down without comment or discussion.

Abbatt and McMahon (1993) identify four distinct phases of the brainstorming exercise. If learning is to take place, the teacher must be clear about what he or she is trying to achieve.

### Phase 1

This involves the need for the group to be clear on the type of idea they are being asked to produce. Examples might include:

- What are the advantages and disadvantages of using the lecture as a teaching method?

- What factors might encourage a patient to stop smoking?

### Phase 2

The facilitator (teacher or student) asks the group for suggestions, and then writes them on the board as quickly as possible. No idea is excluded from the exercise, regardless of how irrelevant it may appear. By the same token, ideas should be recorded even if they have been previously suggested. No comment, judgement or discussion is entered into at this stage.

### Phase 3

All suggestions are examined to ensure that there is a common understanding within the group of all the issues raised, and also to dispense with any ideas that the group feels inappropriate or does not wish to discuss.

### Phase 4

All remaining ideas are then discussed fully, and used to resolve the problem.

Brainstorming is very useful in enabling individual students to increase their confidence within the group. The speed at which the activity is undertaken does not allow the student to consider how his or her idea will be received by the rest of the group, and also enables students further to develop someone else's idea.

Snowballing involves the initial discussion of a subject in small groups, which then develops into a discussion in larger groups (just like a snowball that increases in size as it is rolled). This method has the added advantage that it can be used in larger groups of up to 32 students, as long as space is available.

The process starts with a clear statement of what is wanted from the group – for example, how can we help to ensure patients' and their visitors' personal safety while they are in hospital? Time is then given for each student to think about the issues individually. Their ideas are then combined with those of another student. Between them, they identify the similarities and differences in their ideas and what, if anything, they wish to reject. The pairs then snowball into groups of four, eight and finally 16, during which the issues are compared and discussed until a comprehensive answer is reached.

This is a particularly useful exercise if you are teaching a controversial subject (for example the banning of smoking in all public places), as one group may have to persuade another that their ideas are the 'right' ones.

With buzz groups, students are divided into small groups of between two and six, and each is asked to discuss issues for a short period of time. An appointed reporter (often called a rapporteur) then feeds the information back to the group as a whole. To use the effects of smoking on health as an example, one group could be asked what the physical effects would be, one group the social effects, and so on.

Project presentation is a useful method to use if the subject you are teaching involves the discovery of information. For example, it may be about the function of a voluntary organisation that has been set up to support patients, or about drawing up a community profile. Students can work either singly or in groups. The information gained is presented and shared with the whole of the group, usually using audiovisual equipment.

The methods discussed so far are extremely useful in helping the quieter members of the group to grow in confidence, and in helping them to develop their interpersonal skills.

All of the above have two crucial elements that you, as the teacher, need to consider. First, the purpose of the session should be clear to the students, and second, the students should feel comfortable and safe enough to contribute – for example, they should not feel that they are going to be made to look foolish in front of the group. There is undoubtedly an art in facilitating discussion groups that enables the teacher to support and get the best out of the students. This comes largely with experience.

A seminar is particularly student-centred, as it involves the student presenting either a paper or an essay, following which a group discussion takes place. It is a useful method for exploring sociological issues – for example, the effects of social class on health, or ethical decision-making. Whereas you as a teacher need a sound understanding of the subject material, it is useful to ask the student to formulate two or three questions from the presented paper which can then be discussed by the group.

**ACTIVITY 3.18**   What aspects of teaching from your particular area of practice do you think would be best taught using the group discussion methods?

Role-play is extremely useful in developing problem-solving skills and communication strategies, and in trying to change students' attitudes. It involves students playing the part of other people in a situation previously identified by the teacher. Jarvis (1988) has argued that role-play encourages active participation, enables problems of human behaviour and relationships to be presented, and helps students to understand the relationship between the way in which they think and that in which they feel. It is believed that, because the students have a clearer understanding of themselves, it makes them more aware of the 'roles' adopted by the patients and clients in their care.

However, the use of role-play as a teaching method has been criticised as being unreal (Munroe et al. 1983). The problems enacted may be artificial representations of real events, and students may exaggerate the roles so that they bear little resemblance to reality.

| **ACTIVITY 3.19** | Think about your own learning experiences. Have you taken part in a role-play exercise? If so, did you find the experience enjoyable? If not, why do you think that was? |
|---|---|

You may have found the experience stressful for many reasons. First, the fact that you were required to 'act' in front of the group may have been quite daunting. Second, you were required to 'make it up as you went along'; and third, you may have been asked to enact a role that you had difficulty in relating to. I was once asked to take on the role of a Minister of War. As someone totally opposed to violence, I had some difficulty! It is therefore of vital importance when planning a role-play exercise that the students are comfortable with the process and that you, as a teacher, are sensitive to their needs. It may also be that the method does not meet the student's individual learning style, as identified in earlier chapter.

There are some key steps you may wish to take when planning your role-play:

- Identify clearly what you want the students to learn from the exercise.

- Provide the students with clear guidelines on the character each is to play, and his or her background.

- Keep the situation relatively simple, with no more than four players. If the situation is too complex the teacher can miss some important issues when he or she comes to summarise.

- Give the role players time for preparation.

- Explain clearly to the audience the purpose of the session.

- Explore with the group the key issues raised in the role-play.

The following is an example of role-play and how it may assist learning. This scenario could be used to teach students the communication skills required when faced with behaviour that is difficult to deal with in practice.

A woman telephones the ward and demands to know why her admission has been cancelled. She is extremely angry.

The information given to student A would be as follows: You are a 55-year-old woman who has been on the waiting list for 9 months to have your gall-bladder removed. You are frequently in a great deal of pain. You have just opened your morning's post to discover that the operation you were due to have the day after tomorrow has been cancelled for the second time. This is despite the fact that you contacted the ward yesterday to confirm that it would go ahead, and as a result you have reorganised your work commitments.

The information given to student B would be: You are in charge on a very busy surgical ward. The student nurse comes to tell you there is a lady on the phone who is very angry. The student says it seems that the lady was expecting to be admitted to the ward tomorrow for an operation, which has been cancelled, and wants to know what is going on.

A seemingly simple situation can provide rich opportunities for exploring different strategies for developing communication skills.

Learning from critical incidents is often used in the classroom in order to develop reflective practice. Smith and Russell (1991) provide an excellent example of the application of reflective practice to the teaching situation that involved the use of a journal:

> Everyone was very busy. Sister told me to take [a patient's] wife a cup of tea and sit with her; the doctor would see her shortly. [The wife] didn't know her husband had died. I felt sick. Mrs X asked me how her husband was. I kept saying I didn't know what had happened, but that the doctor would come soon and let her know. I was frightened she would know I was lying. I wished the doctor would hurry (p. 289).

This experience was then used in the classroom to discuss issues relating to communication, the care of people who are dying and their relatives, and stress in nursing.

**ACTIVITY 3.20**    It is likely that in the past you have been taught using the self-directed/independent method. How useful did you find this in terms of your own learning? If you did not find that the method helped you to learn, why was this?

Based on your own experience, you will have your own views about self-directed or independent learning. There are a variety of views on its appropriateness as a teaching method.

There are two key elements to self-directed/independent learning that must be acknowledged if learning is to be effective:

- Students take increasing responsibility for achieving the learning objectives or outcomes.
- Students work at their own pace.

Fundamental to self-directed study is the need for adequate facilities – for example the use of a comprehensive library and information technology. Most criticisms directed at this approach to learning centre on the lack of resources. This is not always the case, however, and entire programmes of study are increasingly being developed in this way. The level of student independence is largely determined by the course planners, who identify what is to be learned and how.

In view of this, there are degrees of self-directed/independent learning. Ewan and White (1996, p. 97) provide a very useful table that identifies stages in the transition from learning being totally teacher-directed to being totally student-directed. It is recognised that courses leading to a nationally recognised qualification are rarely totally self-directed. This is particularly so in pre-registration courses in nursing, largely because of the criteria set down by the statutory bodies in order to maintain standards and patient safety.

**ACTIVITY 3.21** Think about your current role. Make a list of the activities that you think could be taught wholly self-directed, partly self-directed, or wholly teacher-directed.

Self-directed learners become more experienced in working without close supervision. When they enter their jobs as nurses, they are more confident of their own abilities and do not have to rely on someone else to tell them what to do (Ewan and White 1996, p. 98).

Ewan and White say that teachers have a responsibility to help students recognise the importance of what they can contribute to their own and other students' learning. It is important that you try to achieve this in your own teaching. It can be enhanced by:

- Knowing your students well

- Treating them with respect

- Helping them to identify their own learning needs

- Acknowledging that you value their views

- Trying to ensure adequate resources.

Experiential learning plays a key role in learning for many health professionals. In nursing, it is likely that much of your students' learning is experiential.

Experiential learning, according to Burnard (1990), contains five key elements:

- There is an emphasis on personal experience

- It is an active process

- Students are encouraged to reflect on, and therefore learn from, their own experiences

- Experience is valued as a learning episode in itself

- The facilitator/teacher adopts a supportive role in the learning process.

It is clear from the above that the prime place for this type of learning to occur is in practice.

**ACTIVITY 3.22**    How can you, as a practitioner, facilitate experiential learning by students whom you have been allocated? What factors do you think are important?

You have probably identified factors such as your own current knowledge and experience, the time available within your current role to support the student, and your knowledge of what the student already knows. It is important at this stage to note that, whereas curricula in nurse education combine theory and practice, the theory does not always come before the practice: students can learn equally well by gaining some of their experience in practice, and then learning the theory that underpins it. For example, it is possible for a student to be able to undertake a blood pressure recording safely without having a full understanding of the theory relating to hypertension.

# AUDIOVISUAL AIDS

There are many types of aid to help you in your teaching. First, it is useful to identify their value and purpose. Audiovisual aids and technology have several functions. They:

- Enhance the clarity of whatever you are trying to communicate

- Provide diversity in teaching methods

- Aid retention

- Give impact

- Simulate real-life situations

- Permit practice, and thus give confidence

- Use a range of senses

- Increase and sustain attention

- Provide realism

- Increase the meaningfulness of abstract concepts.

Most colleges of nursing have their own information technology or audio-visual department, able to offer specific advice. Although the following list is not exhaustive, it will provide you with an overview of what is available:

- Powerpoint

- Chalkboards (it is worth remembering that these are not easy to write on if you have never practised)

- Whiteboards (remember to use the correct markers that can be erased)

- Felt and magnetic boards

- Interactive videos/computerised programmes

- Charts and models

- Broadcasts

- Tape-recordings

- Films

- Slide projectors.

When deciding whether to use an audiovisual aid, remember that it should not be used as an optional extra – or as the provider of the whole of the teaching that is to take place.

There are some fundamental questions to ask yourself before you make a final decision about the sort of audiovisual aid you want to use. Indeed, there are many other ways of helping students to retain information – for example field trips, which are often an extremely enjoyable way of learning. It is crucial, however, that any visit is relevant to the learning and the theory that underpins it. For example, students at an early point in their studies gain tremendous benefit from discussing the concepts of primary health care in the college setting, and then following this up by a guided tour around a local health centre. The experience must be meaningful for the student if learning is to take place.

If your choice of teaching method is a lesson or lecture, powerpoint or overhead transparencies are a very useful aid to the session. Their use can clarify the key points for students, and assist them to make notes. They have an added advantage for the nervous teacher, in that their use diverts students' attention from the teacher to the screen. There are some basic rules to follow in the preparation and use of powerpoint or overhead transparencies:

- Always use letters at least 1 cm high.

- Never use ordinary typewritten copy: on transparencies it is far too small for anyone sitting beyond the front row to see.

- If you are preparing transparencies by hand, always use a strong base colour   for example, black and blue show up clearly. Red is difficult to see on an overhead projector. Note that some projectors enable you to draw diagrams as you speak.

- Always switch off the projector between uses, and when you have finished. It is not only a strain on the eyes but also an assault on the ears of students, particularly when older machinery is being used.

- Never put too many words on the powerpoint or the transparency. Six lines is probably the maximum for it not to look crowded.

- Resist the temptation to talk to the powerpoint or projector and ignore the students.

- Reveal information one point at a time. This will prevent students from writing everything down before they have had a chance to assimilate the information you are presenting.

- If you cover part of a transparency with a sheet of paper, use a coin to weight the paper down. You will still be able to read the words on the transparency.

- Never put all of your teaching material on powerpoint or transparencies. Not only is it very boring for students, but it will also make your teaching stilted and unspontaneous. Furthermore, the students will be exhausted.

- Give students time to write notes. Remember, a minute of silence is a long time for you, but not for the student who is trying to copy what you have written.

- Provide evidence for what you are saying.

Finally, always have a back-up plan of action. You may need this if the computer or projector light bulb fails. In order to save students from having to copy down what is on your powerpoint or transparencies, you may want to prepare handouts of the content. If all goes well these can be given out at the end. However, in the event of faulty equipment, you can use the handouts as a framework for your session. Remember, if you do prepare handouts, tell the students at the start of the class that these are available to save them trying to copy everything down.

## CONCLUSION

This chapter has focused on factors that have a bearing on the ways in which we learn, and how we can maximise learning in our own working environment. The fact that teaching and learning are closely linked will also influence the way in which we teach, in either the classroom or the practice setting. The chapter has also provided you with the basic information that you will need in order for you to teach effectively, either in your area of practice or in the classroom. It is not intended that the chapter provide you with an in-depth knowledge of the process of teaching and learning, but it should act as a reference point to get you started.

## REFERENCES

Abbatt F, McMahon R. Teaching healthcare workers: a practical guide, 2nd edn. London: Macmillan, 1993

Baldwin A. One-to-one. New York: Evans & Co., 1977

Beitz M. Dynamics of effective oral presentations: strategies for nurse educators. AORN Journal 1994; 59: 1026–1032

Bernstein B. Linguistic codes, hesitation phenomena and intelligence. Language and Speech 1962; 5: 15–17

Bloom BS. Taxonomy of educational objectives. London: Longman, 1972

Boud D, Keogh R, Walker D. Reflections: training experience into learning. London: Kogan Page, 1985

Burnard P. Learning human skills: an experimental guide for nurses, 2nd edn. Oxford: Butterworth-Heinemann, 1990

Burrel T. Curriculum design and development. London: Prentice Hall, 1988

Clifford C. The role of nurse teachers: concerns, conflicts and challenges. Nurse Education Today 1995; 15: 11–16

Concise Oxford Dictionary, 10th edn. United States: Oxford University Press, 1999

Cooper SS. Teaching tips: some lecturing dos and donts. Journal of Continuing Education in Nursing 1989; 20: 140–141

Curzio J. A plan for introducing evidence based practice. Nursing Times 1997; 93: 55–56

Curzon LB. Teaching in further education: an outline of principles and practice, 5th edn. London: Cassell, 1997

Dewing J. Reflective practice. Senior Nurse 1990; 10: 26–28

Ewan C, White R. Teaching nursing: a self instructional handbook, 2nd edn. London: Chapman & Hall, 1996

Ghaye T. An introduction to learning through critical reflective practice. Newcastle upon Tyne: Pentaxion, 1996

Hamer S, Collinson G. Achieving evidence-based practice: a handbook for practitioners: London: Harcourt Brace, 1999

Hudson L. Frames of mind, ability, perception and self perception in the arts and sciences. London: Methuen, 1968

Jarvis P. Adult and continuing education – theory and practice. London: Routledge, 1988

Jolly U. The first-year nurse tutor: a qualitative study. Salisbury: Mark Allen, 1997

Kiger AM. Teaching for health, 2nd edn. New York: Churchill Livingstone, 1995

Knowles M. Androgogy in action. San Francisco: Jossey Bass, 1984

Maslow AH. Motivation and personality. London: Harper & Row, 1987

Mead GH. Mind, self and society. Chicago: University of Chicago Press, 1934

Munroe EA, Manthei R, Small JJ. Counselling skills approach. New Zealand: Methuen, 1983

Nicklin PJ, Kenworthy N. Teaching and assessing in nursing practice: an experiential approach, 3rd edn. London: Harcourt Brace, 2000

Nursing and Midwifery Council. Code of professional conduct. London, 2002

Osler W. In: Daintith J, Isaacs A. Medical quotations. Collins reference dictionary. Glasgow: Market House Books, 1989; p. 200

Parkin C. Humor, health, and higher education: laughing matters. Journal of Nurse Education 1989; 28: 229–230

Pask G. Styles and strategies of learning. British Journal of Educational Psychology 1976; 46: 128–148

Prognoff I. Journal workshop. New York: Dialogue House Library, 1975

Quinn FM. The principles and practice of nurse education, 4th edn. Cheltenham: Thornes, 2000

Rogers C. Freedom to learn for the 80s. Columbus OH: Charles E Merrill, 1983

Sargent A. Turning people on: the motivation challenge. London: Institute of Personnel Management, 1990

Skinner BF. The technology of teaching. New York: Appleton-Century-Croft, 1968

Smith A, Russell J. Using critical learning: incidents in nurse education. Nurse Education Today 1991; 11: 284–291

Stengelhofen J. Teaching students in clinical settings. London: Chapman & Hall, 1996

United Kingdom Central Council for Nurses Midwives and Health Visitors. Post Registration Education and Practice Project. London: UKCC, 1994

Wallace M. Lifelong learning: PREP in action. Edinburgh: Harcourt Brace, 1999

Welsh I, Swann C. Partners in learning: a guide to support and assessment in nurse education. Oxford: Radcliffe Medical Press, 2002

# FURTHER READING

*The following books provide further information on the theories of learning and the practice of teaching. Both use a logical framework.*

Hergenhahn BR. An introduction to theories of learning, 5th edn. London: Prentice Hall International, 1997

Jarvis P. The theory and practice of teaching. London: Kogan Page, 2002

# 4 Teaching for competency-based learning

*Anne Eaton and Sue Hinchliff*

---

## INTRODUCTION

This chapter explores the notion of competence in nursing practice. This concept is gaining in importance in today's NHS, with the pay modernisation agenda being focused on the NHS Knowledge and Skills Framework and all the issues regarding competencies being attached to roles. Preparation for initial practice is now firmly competency-based, and here we look at how competencies can form a part of professional accreditation at post-registration level.

## LEARNING OBJECTIVES

After reading this chapter you should be able to:

- Give an overview of what is meant by competence
- Describe the NHS Knowledge and Skills Framework

◆ Relate this to appraisal and personal development plans

◆ Differentiate between academic and professional accreditation

◆ Identify three types of model for accreditation

◆ Recognise the benefits of professional accreditation

◆ Distinguish standards from competencies

◆ Determine the stages in the process of professional accreditation.

## OVERVIEW OF COMPETENCE

The World Health Organization described competence as requiring: 'knowledge and appropriate attitudes and observable mechanical and intellectual skills which together account for the ability to deliver a specific professional service' (WHO 1998).

Another definition is that of the International Council of Nurses which, in 1997, defined competence as 'a level of performance demonstrating the effective application of knowledge, skill and judgement' (ICN 1997).

The definition of competence that was applied to pre-registration nursing programmes leading to professional registration by the erstwhile United Kingdom Central Council (UKCC 1999) is: 'the skills and ability to practice safely and effectively without the need for direct supervision'.

When looking at these definitions it appears that key words are common, though not consistent throughout the definitions; these key words are:

● Skills

● Ability

● Knowledge

● Attitudes.

**ACTIVITY 4.1**    Devise your own definition of competence, perhaps for a specific group of learners, or as a generic statement covering all learners.

It might be useful here to remind you of such a generic statement developed by Storey et al., who attempted to capture these key words:

Competence is the knowledge, skills, abilities and behaviours that a practitioner needs to perform their work to a professional standard, and is a key lever for achieving results that will enable the organisation to achieve its health care objectives' (Storey et al. 2002).

We have already looked at some competence-based programmes and frameworks, namely pre-registration nursing programmes and the NVQ/SVQ framework. This chapter concentrates on the National Health Service Knowledge and Skills Framework (NHS KSF) developed as part of the NHS modernisation agenda throughout 2001 and 2002. This was implemented in 'Early Implementor Sites' (EIS) in England throughout 2003, and will be integrated throughout the whole of the NHS and the UK from 2004 onwards.

**What is the NHS KSF?**

The NHS KSF has been developed as a shared initiative between representatives from health service unions, health service managers and Department of Health staff. The development and ultimate use of the NHS KSF has been based on the following principles (DoH 2003):

- Simple, easy to explain and understand

- Operationally feasible to implement

- Able to use and link with current and emerging competence frameworks

- NHS-wide

- Supportive of the delivery of plans for the future development of the NHS in the four countries of the UK.

Following on from these principles is the notion that the NHS KSF has been designed to:

- Identify the knowledge and skills that individuals need to apply in their posts

- Help guide the development of individuals

- Provide a fair and objective framework on which to base review and development for all staff.

These aims have been developed bearing in mind, and with reference to, previous work in all four countries of the UK, including the NHS Plan for England in 2000 and *Our National Health: a Plan for Action, a Plan for Change*, produced by the Scottish Executive in 2000.

Reading this you may already be asking questions about the feasibility of such a major undertaking, which covers the whole of the NHS (except medical staff) across all four UK countries – and the NHS being one of the largest employers in the UK. This is indeed an ambitious undertaking and will not happen overnight, but will be integrated throughout this massive organisation over a substantial period of time. The reason for this delay is the infrastructure that will need to be developed to support its implementation.

Remember that the NHS KSF will cover all NHS staff – not just nurses, not just allied health care professionals, but everyone, including porters, catering staff, cleaning staff, and grounds staff, to name but a few. Some of these staff groups will have had little if any personal development, other than mandatory updates in such areas as fire safety or health and safety at work.

**ACTIVITY 4.2**   List as many members of staff as you can whom you come across as part of your normal working practices in your role. Your answers might include:

- Nurses
- HCAs
- Doctors
- Physiotherapists
- Occupational therapists
- Speech and language therapists
- Ward receptionists
- Phlebotomists
- Porters
- Radiographers
- Radiologists
- Operating department practitioners
- Catering staff
- Dietitians
- Cleaners.

And on and on and on!!

The NHS KSF will be used to identify the competence of individuals in their posts and will then be used in appraisal and development reviews, and in the application and development of personal development plans (PDP), which all staff will be expected to create, apply and develop.

Some groups, including nurses, undertake this process now in the context of continuing professional development and post-registration education and practice (PREP). However, for other groups this is a daunting proposition and will need skilful and dedicated support if it is to work in the way it has been envisaged.

Effective development of the initiative will be characterised by a partnership approach between employers – or managers acting on their behalf – and individual members of staff. As a partnership approach both parties need to take responsibility for fulfilling their agreed roles. You may be asking why we need this process when we have managed without it so far. Before we come to that, perhaps you can begin to answer it yourself by looking at your answer to the activity above and considering the staff you have not listed as well as the staff you have! The public – i.e. patients and clients receiving care within the NHS – are confused by the plethora of staff with different job titles and similar roles, and by the fragmented nature of the care they receive.

**ACTIVITY 4.3**

Try to work through the scenario of a patient attending surgical outpatients for the first time, and list the departments and staff they may be exposed to. Your answers might include:

- GP/practice nurse in the first instance, who referred them to the surgeon
- Receptionist – booked them in for their appointment
- Health care assistant (HCA) – did baseline observations of blood pressure, weight, height, urinalysis etc.
- Nurse – took them into the consulting room and prepared them for the consultant
- Medical student/junior doctor who took medical history
- Consultant surgeon
- Receptionist in X-ray department
- Radiographer, or clinical imaging nurse
- Phlebotomist – a variety of blood samples.

**ACTIVITY 4.4**

Can you plan a better service for patients moving through this process, perhaps with a 'one stop shop' in mind?

These activities stemmed from the question – Why do we need the NHS KSF? The answer is that we ultimately need to improve the quality of services to patients across the NHS. So, the purpose of the NHS KSF, linked to development reviews, is to:

- Promote equality for all staff – with every member of staff (except doctors) using the same framework, having the same opportunities for learning and development open to them, and having the same structured learning, development and review. *This learning presupposes that there are practitioners out there who are able and willing to support this learning – which is where you come in!*

- Promote effectiveness at work – with managers and staff being clear about what is required within a role and how an individual can be more effective through the provision of appropriate learning and development opportunities

- Support effective learning and development of individuals and teams – with all members of staff being supported to learn throughout their careers and develop in a variety of ways, and being given the resources to do so.

It is necessary here to introduce you to the NHS KSF so that you can begin to gain an understanding of the process. Essentially the NHS KSF is a development tool. It is made up of a number of dimensions, six of which have been identified as core to all NHS staff and roles – these dimensions occur in everyone's job. A further 16 dimensions have been developed, and it is envisaged that only a small number of these will apply to each individual – no role will cover all of the specific dimensions, as they have been developed to be job specific. Although all of the dimensions are listed in numerical order this does not imply a hierarchy: the numbering system has been used purely to aid easy recognition and referencing, and the potential development of a computer-based tool.

The dimensions are then divided into level descriptors, which show increasingly advanced knowledge and skill and complexity of application of knowledge and skills to the demands of work. So, unlike the system for the dimensions, the process through the levels *is* incremental, and an individual cannot claim to be working at a specific level within the descriptors of a dimension without demonstrating their competence in the other, lower-level descriptors.

The next breakdown within the dimensions is that each level descriptor then has attached to it:

- **Indicators**   These describe the level at which knowledge and skills need to be applied, and they have been designed so as to enable more consistent and reliable application of the dimensions and descriptors across the NHS.

- **Examples of applications**   These have been devised and included to illustrate how, and to what, the dimensions, level descriptors and indicators could be applied across the jobs within the NHS. These examples relate generically to all jobs, and specifically in relation to a particular area of work or a specific technology.

- **References**   These signpost users to further information and connections to the KSF, and these references include regulatory competences, perhaps attached to continuing professional development (CPD) criteria, National Occupational Standards, other nationally developed competences, and national guidance.

Many NHS employers and Trusts have developed their own competence frameworks over the last few years, some of which are occupation specific and some of which are generic.

The only competence frameworks that have been referenced within the NHS KSF are those that have been nationally developed and quality assured through some national mechanism, for example National Occupational Standards. However, employers can 'bolt on' their competence framework to the KSF – in effect, putting some local detail on to what are the bare bones of the NHS KSF. This is vitally important, as the NHS KSF is about the development of individuals and roles, and that is exactly what an employer can achieve by marrying the two frameworks. What must not happen is that individuals are required to produce evidence for two or more functions in different ways. The evidence produced should meet the demands of NHS KSF, the local competence framework, and CPD demands for a professional with *one* portfolio of evidence (see later in the chapter).

So, let us return to look at the content of the NHS KSF.

# NHS KSF CORE DIMENSIONS

Remember, these have been developed to match every single role and therefore every individual within the NHS except doctors. The core dimensions are:

1. Communication

2. Personal and people development

3. Health, safety and security

4. Service development

5. Quality

6. Equality, diversity and rights.

## Specific dimensions

Remember that these are designed to fit specific roles, and therefore no individual will fulfil all of the specific dimensions: rather, they will match their role to what will be a small number of specific dimensions. These are:

7. Assessment of health and well-being needs

8. Addressing individuals' health and well-being needs

9. Promotion of health and well-being

10. Protection of health and well-being

11. Logistics

12. Data processing and management

13. Production and communication of information and knowledge

14. Facilities maintenance and management

15. Design and production of equipment, devices and visual records

16. Biomedical investigation and reporting

17. Application of technology for measurement, monitoring and treatment

18. Partnership

19. Leadership

20. Management of people

21. Management of physical and financial resources

22. Research and development.

**ACTIVITY 4.5**

Although you only have the titles of the dimensions above, try to match your role within the core and specific dimensions, and then match the role of one of your learners to the NHS KSF dimensions (not a nursing student, as they will not be involved with the NHS KSF until they are qualified nurses – remember that as nursing students they are not employed by the NHS).

For yourself as a qualified nurse, for example, you might place yourself within all of the core dimensions and within specific dimensions numbers 7, 8 and 9.

For an HCA, for example, you might have again recognised all of the core dimensions and matched them to specific dimensions 7 and 8.

Alarm bells may now be ringing for you as you ask yourself what is the difference between yourself as a registered professional and HCAs working in support of you. The answer lies in the level descriptors!

Let's illustrate this issue by looking at one dimension which is seen to be common to you and to the HCA, dimension number 7 – Assessment of health and well-being needs.

When we look at the descriptors to this dimension we see there are four levels, which are incremental in nature:

● Level 1 – assist in assessing individuals' health and well-being needs

● Level 2 – assess the health and well-being needs of people whose needs are relatively stable and consistent with others in the caseload

- Level 3 – assess the health and well-being needs of people whose needs are complex and change across the workload
- Level 4 – develop practice in the assessment of health and well-being needs.

Remember that these descriptors are then further broken down into indicators, so an indicator for descriptor 1 might be: 'provides accurate information to the team on the support that individuals will need and the impact of this on his/her own work'. Likewise, an example of an indicator at level 4 might be: follows processes of reasoning which:

- Balance additional information against the overall picture of the individual's needs to confirm or deny developing hypotheses
- Are capable of justification given the available information at the time
- Are likely to result in the optimum outcome.

Now you can see that the descriptors are incremental. When you revisit the activity above, you might identify that the specific dimensions are the same, but for dimension 7, for example, you as a professional practitioner might fit dimension 3 and your HCA fits dimension 1, hence the difference in roles between the professional and the non-professional in this example.

You might be wondering how this all fits within the context of this book. A substantial amount of teaching and learning will be needed for individuals to recognise, acknowledge and achieve the needs of the NHS KSF to support their learning and the provision of evidence to demonstrate that they can meet their target dimensions and descriptors.

Before we look at this you need to make the link between the NHS KSF and development review and the use of personal development plans.

## DEVELOPMENT REVIEW

Development review is a cyclical process of review, planning, development and evaluation for all staff in the NHS, linked to organisational and individual needs. In the past this has been more popularly termed appraisal, but this tended to apply only to professional or managerial positions and was rarely used for other staff. Within the NHS KSF the development review will be a partnership between an individual member of staff and their manager, or someone acting in that capacity. Remember that from your perspective you may not only be the one undergoing a development review: you may also be the manager supporting others through their review. Whoever is undertaking the review must be competent to do so. This means that managers and others need to develop these skills, and this may well include developing their knowledge and understanding of the roles and jobs of individual staff members. One of the aims of the NHS KSF is to develop all staff, and therefore an intended outcome of this framework is to ensure that resources of all kinds are available so that all staff can progress and develop to meet the knowledge and skills of their current post and to progress through their career pathways should they choose to do so.

The main aim of the development review process is to:

- Review how individuals are applying their knowledge and skills to meet the demands of their current position

- Identify the development needs of the member of staff

- Identify the development needs that a person has over a given period of time

- Plan how and where this development will take place and agree the date of the next review.

Stop here for a moment and revisit the content of Chapter 3, where teaching and learning in practice was detailed. Teaching and learning are an integral part of development. As a practitioner you may find that you are both the teacher and the learner, or in the context of development reviews within the NHS KSF the reviewer and the reviewee!

The review cycle is not new: it has been part of education in general and nurse education in particular for a considerable time. Indeed, Kolb (1993) termed this the adult learning cycle, which has four stages:

1. A joint review between the individual and their line manager (or, in the context of the NHS KSF, another person acting as the manager) matched and plotted against the demands of the post and any other agreed targets

2. The production of a PDP which identifies the learning and development needs of the individual, including short- and long-term aims and an agreement as to how these aims are going to be facilitated and achieved

3. Undertaking the learning and development planned by the individual

4. An evaluation of the learning and development that has occurred, including the application of this learning.

Stage 4 completes the cycle but also starts it again; development is not a static process, nor is it done only once – progression and development are ongoing. Even for those members of staff who do not wish to progress further, there is still the issue of maintaining their knowledge and skills in order to 'stand still'. Care needs and care delivery is never static: new processes and technologies are constantly being developed and all staff need to keep abreast of new developments in order to maintain the same competent delivery, whatever their role may be.

For registered professionals, including nurses, this is not a new process, although here it may seem more prescriptive than CPD to meet the needs of PREP. A reminder here for all registered nurses – and also to any individual who needs to demonstrate their CPD to their employer or regulatory body – that evidence collected for their NHS KSF development plan and contained in a portfolio can also be used for their regulatory CPD and re-registration needs, and indeed for any situation that demands evidence of their role and competence.

---

**ACTIVITY 4.6**

List areas of your professional life where evidence may be needed to demonstrate knowledge and skills – or competence. Your answers might include:

- PREP
- NHS KSF
- Induction
- Promotion
- Job interview
- Application to an academic programme
- Accreditation of prior experiential learning (APEL).

---

As we can see from this list it makes sense to have one portfolio that fits many needs. I am not suggesting here that the evidence for one need automatically fits the evidence for another, but that with some rearrangement – which might include adding or taking away specific pieces of evidence – one portfolio can fit many purposes!

Readers might be asking why a development review is necessary. If so, think back to when you wanted to progress or demonstrate your knowledge and skills to your manager. You probably did not have information easily to hand; we need development reviews so that the individual will benefit from the process by:

- Having clear expectations of the demands of the post and support from their manager to meet those expectations

- Managers taking a focused interest in your work, your development and your learning, based on an explicit and objective knowledge and skills framework

- Having available resources to support learning and development.

So, development reviews are not new for some members of the care environment, and they should not pose a threat or a demand for yet more bureaucracy or paperwork. Their complexity will vary according to the role and needs of the individual member of staff. Development – or at least the maintenance of current levels of knowledge and skills – needs to be a high priority for managers and employers alike, in order to deliver the best possible care to patients and clients.

Before leaving this section, perhaps it is worth looking at exactly what is a PDP. A PDP is the outcome of the planning stage of the development review process – it simply plans development for the individual! Although the needs of the employer and the organisation need to be included in the PDP it is not exclusive to these areas. As this is a personal development plan, there should be something in it that relates to the development of the person concerned as an individual, and not merely as an employee. Personal interests and opportunities for progression ought to be included, and a well-developed PDP will strike a comfortable balance between the needs of the employer and those of the individual.

## LINKING THE DEVELOPMENT REVIEW WITH THE NHS KSF

In the first instance, even before the development review takes place, the manager and the individual staff member need to be clear about the expectations of that individual within their current post. This is done by developing a KSF outline for that post, or by matching the current post against the generic and specific dimensions and descriptors of the KSF. This outline will usually be carried out by the manager and the human resources department. It may involve the postholder and other parties, for example if it is a joint appointment with two different stakeholders involved. Remember that it is the post that is being matched against the KSF, and not the individual who holds the post. Once the KSF outline has been developed then this is matched against the individual who holds the post, to determine whether or not they are functioning well in that post. This part of the review might show that the individual exceeds the outline in some of the dimensions identified, but it may also show that some areas are not strong and that the individual fails to achieve the dimensions and descriptors outlined for the post.

So, a development need is recognised and a plan is drawn up for how this need will be met, by when, and what resources are needed; in other words, a learning contact will be developed and agreed, in order to enable the individual to reach the desired dimension and descriptor. Remember that the review should identify short- and long-term goals, so that priorities will be identified and met.

For someone new in post this is a relatively easy process, but for existing staff it raises questions that need to be agreed on an individual basis. It might seem appropriate to start to develop job descriptions for posts, based on the dimensions and descriptors of the NHS KSF – at least then they will be based on national standards and appear consistent across all employers.

Once a PDP has been developed it is worth looking at ways in which this learning and development can be facilitated.

**ACTIVITY 4.7**   List the methods you can think of for facilitating learning and development.

You may have suggested a number of options, which might include:

- Formal courses
- Role-play
- Learning sets
- Induction programmes
- Distance learning
- Private study
- e-learning
- Reflective practice
- Participating in specific areas of work
- Learning from others on the job
- Experiential learning.

**ACTIVITY 4.8**   Which methods would suit your learning needs best? Which methods do you prefer to incorporate in your teaching?

You might have listed similar processes for both situations, but you need to think about not only your preferred methods of teaching but also whether these methods meet the needs of your learners.

## ACCREDITATION

We will now move on to look at accreditation, which is one means of developing, as a practitioner can become accredited at differing levels of competence within his or her role.

Professional accreditation differs significantly in its focus from academic accreditation, which is usually called validation. Academic accreditation ensures that an educational initiative (a course or a module) is fit for purpose and fit for an award. It focuses on issues such as a relevant and up-to-date curriculum, the students' experience of the course, teaching strategies, how quality is monitored, the academic environment etc. Academic accreditation is to do with the learning experience, and it is the educational initiative that is accredited.

In nursing professional accreditation focuses first and foremost on patient/client-centred care and on fitness for practice, and can include:

- How knowledge is used in practice to improve care
- How professional competence is developed, maintained and measured
- Ways in which practice standards are met
- The development and use of professional judgement
- Effective use of the interprofessional health care team
- The environment and culture of care etc.

In essence, professional accreditation focuses on how people, products or places influence nursing practice and patient/client care. It is about what happens in practice – and methods based in practice are used to assess whether a person or place can be awarded professional accreditation.

Both professional and academic accreditation share a common principle i.e. *they are both based on a judgement by peers about compliance with a set of standards (or competencies) using agreed criteria.* However, they can be differentiated in terms of a number of characteristics. Table 4.1 attempts to capture some of these; it is not exhaustive, but captures some key differences.

Generally models of accreditation are based on the type of standards that are used and there is a continuum, from standards for best practice to minimum standards for safe practice.

- In terms of best practice we are talking about aiming for excellence, with the use of evidence-based practice – upholding the best possible standards of care. The use of optimal standards sets an aspirational level. Note, though, that there is a place here for recognising that there may be constraints that stand in the way of total excellence. Optimum standards can be kite-marked at a point in time ... or an accreditation body can work with people, products or workplaces to develop and shape the person, product or workplace towards being the best. Often this model is used when accreditation is sought voluntarily – it is associated with quality improvement; this is a developmental model.

| TABLE 4.1 | Comparison between academic and professional accreditation | | |
|-----------|------------------------------------------------------------|---|---|
| **Characteristic** | **Academic** | **Professional** |
| Context of the awarding authority | Based in higher education institutions | Based in professional organisations and practice |
| Main focus | Programmes of study/modules Achievement in terms of academic award/credit points Fitness for award | Individual professionals Achievement in terms of professional practice/patient care Fitness for practice |
| Key components | Degree of challenge in terms of level (1, 2, 3 & higher) Effort hours (10 per credit point) National qualifications framework Subject benchmarks | Models of continuing professional development and competence Framework with domains and levels of practice Career and competency framework |
| Nature of assessment | Focus mainly on learning outcomes, assessment-based system, using internal/external examiners | Focus mainly on impact on practice, practitioners and the health care team Portfolio-based Based on triangulation involving evidence from practice External peer reviewed |
| Outcomes | Validated programmes/modules Academic credit awarded | Professional recognition Usually includes certification |

- Minimum standards models are consistent with 'doing the patient no harm' – safe, but not necessarily the best. Rules and regulations are set at this level and no organisation should fall below it. Regulation, too, has to be set at minimum levels of safety, not pitched at levels of excellence. This can be the model used when accreditation is mandatory. It does not add value as such. It can be useful in order to assure a level playing field. In a poor organisation it provides a starting point, anything falling below it being unacceptable. It may also be all that is possible in an emergency. It tends to be associated with inspection.

- A normative model comes somewhere in between the two above, where most organisations should be able to achieve the normative standards that are not pitched at a minimum – nor are they pitched at a level of aspirational excellence.

**ACTIVITY 4.9**

A quick quiz: which of the following apply to accreditation?

- Promotes 'feel-good factor'
- Establishes credibility
- Helps to maintain standards
- Offers a 'kite mark'
- Facilitates continuous review of current practice and its development
- Puts a value on professional nursing
- Makes nursing practice more visible
- Helps to maintain consistency
- Enhances the accreditee's reputation
- Offers a structured framework for innovations in practice
- Provides a basis for collaborative working
- Helps to improve patient care
- Aids recruitment and retention/enhances job satisfaction
- Offers experience of a range of evaluation methodologies
- Uses peer review
- Promotes reflection and support
- Facilitates learning from and in practice.

Well – it didn't take much working out that they all describe the benefits of accreditation! If you didn't get the answer right, maybe you need to know a bit more about professional accreditation.

Professional accreditation is about setting standards and helping practitioners shape their practice towards those standards. It is about helping to maintain consistency throughout service delivery – and it is about taking pride in this.

The value of accreditation depends on where you are standing. The benefits are obviously different, depending on whether you are a practitioner, an employer or a patient or client.

**ACTIVITY 4.10**

Look back over your personal and professional life to an occasion when you were accredited. It might not have been called accreditation – but when you took your driving test (assuming that you have!), for example, you were licensed (accredited) as a driver. When you became registered as a nurse you were accredited – and given a licence to practise. How did it feel? What were the benefits? How were you seen by others?

I am sure that you felt good. You became able to do things that you were not permitted to do before – and you achieved a particular status.

The patient or client always has to be central to whatever we do in accreditation. After all, ensuring best practice in educational initiatives for nurses, in nursing practice and in competency development ultimately improves outcomes for patients and clients. If you were a patient you would feel reassured to know that your primary nurse had been recognised as an expert practitioner;

or that he or she had just undertaken a programme to prepare him or her as an RCN-recognised Clinical Leader. You could be confident that the nurse had achieved certain standards of practice, or had reached particular practice benchmarks. It's a way of knowing that something or someone has measured up – and that's what professional accreditation is all about.

Employers are concerned about value for money, and when offering CPD opportunities to their staff they want to know that the event, short course or resource has been examined against predetermined quality standards and found to be both educationally sound and of appropriate design and content to achieve its purpose. It should also be offered by experts who are recognised as being qualified to teach on the topic. Accreditation is, therefore, a proxy for assuring all these elements.

Employers are also concerned to offer a service that is fit for purpose and fit for practice. Competency development is key to quality improvement, and professional accreditation facilitates a constant review of current practice. Practice development provides a basis for collaborative working and offers a structured framework for developing innovations in practice that ultimately increase staff satisfaction – all of which contribute to improved recruitment and retention of the professional workforce – and so everyone benefits.

What are the benefits, then, to practitioners? Well, for one thing there is a feel-good factor about being accredited – it feels like the achievement it is! It is something to be celebrated; it could be used in a bid for promotion; it establishes credibility in the area that is accredited. At one extreme, being accredited for your expertise in a specialised area of practice is a step on the way to becoming a Consultant Nurse. When a practitioner is accredited as an individual, he or she has to put together a portfolio of evidence of different kinds, demonstrating that the relevant standards have been met. This gives the opportunity to experiment with and experience a range of assessment methodologies, such as 360° reviews, user narratives, direct observation of care, taped or videotaped exchanges, and so on.

Although it is only through academic validation that CATS (Credit Accumulation and Transfer Scheme) points are awarded, the evidence collected for professional accreditation could be submitted to an Institution of Higher Education for APEL in order to gain some exemption from a formal course of study towards an award.

So, if accreditation has a wide range of benefits, what is the downside? Well, accreditation presents a snapshot of a person, educational product or practice area at a particular point in time. In order for that accolade to continue to hold true there must be regular review and performance monitoring, and these should be capable of showing growth and further development.

Nobody would deny that it is time-consuming to develop effective standards. Even then, as practitioners develop and as time moves on, the standards can be pushed further towards excellence. Equally, on the part of the person seeking accreditation it can be a lengthy process to put all the required evidence together. Accreditation is never a quick fix! Those who are to assess evidence must be rigorously prepared, monitored, and continue to be offered development opportunities. For all these reasons, accreditation costs money, but the benefits outweigh those costs. It may also take some time to achieve.

In essence, accreditation – whether for a person, an educational product or a workplace – involves four stages:

- Standard/competency setting
- Dissemination of the standards/competencies with guidance to facilitate the collection of evidence
- Comparison of the evidence against the standards/competencies by peers to ensure compliance
- Review and evaluation of all stages of the foregoing process in order to effect quality enhancement.

## Standard/competency setting

A standard is a desired and achievable level of performance against which actual performance can be measured. It does not tell you what a person can *do*, but it can tell you what a product, person or place should *look like*. The European Union, for instance, has standards about what tomatoes should be like – in terms of size, shape, imperfections etc. The Army has standards about what soldiers should look like in their uniforms.

Competencies refer to the specific knowledge, skills, judgement and personal attributes required for a practitioner to practise safely and ethically in a designated role and setting. One of the characteristics of a self-regulating profession is the development of standards/competencies based on the values of that profession.

Standards and competencies are set by peers who have expertise in the pertinent area of practice. It is usual for educationalists, subject experts, and practice developers to be involved in standard and competency setting. All standards and competencies that are produced should be field-tested before they are put into general use, amended, and then peer reviewed again.

## Dissemination of the standards/competencies

Whatever is being accredited, the applicant requires guidance in the collection of a body of rigorous evidence to support their application for accreditation.

It is the accreditee's responsibility to present this evidence of achievement of the standards or competencies.

## Comparison of the evidence

This is the third stage of accreditation, where peer reviewers check that the person, product or place seeking accreditation can produce evidence to show they/it can meet the standards/competencies. Clearly, it is crucial that all reviewers and staff who play a part in the accreditation process are expert and up-to-date with both their clinical specialism and the accreditation processes.

## Review and evaluation

Each of the above stages should be reviewed on a regular basis, using evaluations from a range of users. Clearly, if changes to effect improvement are to be made, then evaluative comments indicating amendments must be corroborated from a number of sources.

What are the implications of all this for teaching in the clinical area? In a way, it does not matter whether the practitioner is seeking accreditation as a registered nurse (i.e. he or she is a student) or of expertise in practice. The needs for teaching in the clinical area are broadly similar.

To progress their practice competencies practitioners need to gain professional craft knowledge (see Chapter 2). Remember that this arises from a blend of propositional knowledge (all about evidence, research and theory), personal knowledge (from life experience) and professional knowledge (gained over time from practice). Professional craft knowledge or professional mastery is the result.

There is a need to focus on competencies as they arise in practice. There has to be a period of role-modelling, supported practice and supported reflection in and on practice. Clinical supervision, professional facilitation and action learning are key processes to enable practitioners to become more effective and competent. In order to learn this professional craft knowledge one needs other professionals who share one's values and beliefs – and who can offer both challenge and support. It can feel quite risky exposing one's practice to another for critique, and this therefore demands considerable trust on the part of the learner.

The teacher/supervisor/facilitator must (Smith 2001):

- Be an active listener
- Clarify what is discussed and distil its essence

- Identify inconsistencies in ideas, beliefs and actions
- Challenge and confront
- Listen to feelings.

| ACTIVITY 4.11 | Smith (2001) said: |

While limited opportunities still exist for professional development provided by higher education institutions and employing agencies, the most ubiquitous and powerful opportunities for learning lie in the ongoing systematic investigation of daily practice' (p. 176).

Draw up an action plan for working with one practitioner in your clinical area over the next 2 weeks, focusing on how you can help him or her systematically to investigate his or her daily practice. Keep a reflective diary for this period, if you do not already do so, and record your feelings and what you learn from the experience.

## CONCLUSION

At the end of this chapter you should have a sound understanding of competence and how it is being used within the UK health service, and how it links with development reviews, PDPs and professional accreditation. Importantly, you should be able to see where you, as a practitioner/teacher, can contribute to nurses' learning in this area.

## REFERENCES

Department of Health. The NHS Knowledge of Skills Framework (NHS KSF) and development review guidance. Working Draft. DoH, March 2003

International Council of Nurses. ICN on regulation: towards 21st century models. Geneva: ICN, 1997

Kolb D. Experiential learning. New York: Prentice Hall, 1993

Smith D. Facilitating the development of professional craft knowledge. In: Higgs J, Titchen A, eds. Practice knowledge and expertise. Oxford: Butterworth-Heinemann 2001

Storey L, Howard J, Gillies A. Competency in healthcare: a practical guide to competency frameworks. Oxford: Radcliffe Medical Press, 2002

United Kingdom Central Council. Fitness for practice. London: UKCC, 1999

World Health Organization. Learning to work together for health. Report of a WHO study group on multiprofessional education in health personnel: a team approach. Geneva: WHO, 1988

# 5 Evaluating learning and teaching

*Anne Eaton and Sue Howard*

# INTRODUCTION

Throughout this book, reference has been made to the need for continuing professional development across a lifetime of learning, not only to ensure that we provide high-quality patient care, but also to enable us to develop as individuals and meet our own aspirations throughout our careers. Implicit in this journey is the need to know exactly where we are on the path on which we are embarking and, equally importantly, what we need to do to progress along it. This requires us to take time to think about whether where we are going, and what we are teaching and learning, fits with what it is we want to do. In other words, we need to evaluate our progress. This chapter looks at ways in which we can do this.

---

**LEARNING OBJECTIVES**

After reading this chapter you should be able to:

◆ Explain the relationship between evaluation and assessment

◆ Understand the principles underpinning effective student support

◆ Identify and use some of the tools available

◆ Define competence and its relationship to quality patient/client care

◆ Have an understanding of the NVQ/SVQ framework.

---

# DEFINING TERMS

The terms 'assessment' and 'evaluation' are often used interchangeably, yet they are fundamentally different. Ellington et al. (1993) distinguish between the concepts of assessment and evaluation as follows:

- **Assessment** – measures student learning, which is achieved as a result of a teaching/learning situation

- **Evaluation** – is a series of activities that are designed to measure the effectiveness of a teaching/learning system as a whole.

In this chapter the main emphasis, therefore, is on evaluation, as we wish to explore not only what has been taught and subsequently learned, but also to check things out along the way.

Although you are probably undertaking the role of teacher and mentor/assessor in clinical practice, you are also a learner in this situation, and the evaluation processes outlined in the chapter will apply to you in both your teaching and your learning. However, as a teacher you will need to evaluate individually and contribute to the evaluation of the learners in your clinical environment, and you will therefore be evaluating *their* learning.

Assessment can be defined as the collection of data on which we can base evaluation – and assessment can be seen to be descriptive and objective; that is, if another assessor were to undertake the job of assessing the same item, the findings should be the same.

Evaluation could also be seen as the process of making judgements and decisions about achievements, about expectations and about the effectiveness and value of what we are doing. Evaluation involves ideas about 'good' and 'bad' teaching and learning: that is, it relates to its worth, and these ideas are based upon the evaluator's own ideology.

It can be suggested that assessment is value free, objective and, on the whole, criterion referenced – that is, assessment of work using a set of standards or criteria (see Chapter 3). On the other hand, evaluation is a value judgement concept and involves examining and judging the quality, significance, amount, degree or condition of something. In your case, that 'something' will be the processes your learners have gone through and which you have assessed – i.e. your teaching and their learning.

Thus, we can see that the assessment of learners of all kinds forms the major part of any evaluation process, and the outcomes of both should identify not only learning achieved by the individual, but also the educational programme, whether it is delivered in the classroom or the workplace, that fits the purpose. Remember that, as in the nursing process, evaluation is one of four components: assessment, planning, implementation and evaluation. You can apply these components to your role as teacher and assessor.

This does not mean that evaluation occurs only at the end of a learning experience but rather, that it is ongoing and vital to the development and evolution of learning and teaching. The ultimate outcome of evaluation is decision-making, that is, identifying what needs to be changed and changing it. This then leads back into the cycle of activity and on to the assessment of learning needs. The intention of evaluation is to make conscious what most of us do much of the time as part of the process of teaching (Rogers 1994).

Evaluation may be one of the more difficult skills required of you in your role as teacher, and it is important that the techniques involved – and indeed the whole process – are developed consciously.

In your clinical area, and with the many learners you come across in your work activities, there is no point in evaluating your teaching, and the learning that has taken place, if you are not prepared to change what you do as a result of the feedback the evaluation process gives you. Evaluation can only be effective if you are prepared to stop the existing programme when a problem is detected and redevelop both the programme and your teaching accordingly. However, it would be foolhardy and impulsive to act immediately on the results of one evaluation that may identify a relatively minor problem. It is more appropriate to wait and see whether subsequent evaluations give the same results; if so, *then* is the time to change the relevant part of the programme. If action is taken too early, change may be made when it is not necessary. With each successive cycle of evaluation, the processes of teaching and learning should become progressively more refined, and the ultimate results should become more effective and efficient.

In my own experience, I changed my teaching of how to record blood pressure when one learner could not grasp the skill, only to find eventually that the failure in fact laid with the learner. Conversely, I maintained another session because I felt comfortable with it, when it was obvious from learner assessment that very few of the group were learning.

## EVALUATION AS A PROCESS

To develop the notion of evaluating teaching and learning, we need to explore the following questions:

- Why do we need to evaluate?

- When is the best time to evaluate?

- Where is the most appropriate place to evaluate?

- What is it we need to evaluate?

- Who are we going to evaluate?

- How do we evaluate?

## Why do we need to evaluate?

It is important to recognise that evaluation occurs throughout many different levels of the teaching and learning process.

**ACTIVITY 5.1**    From your personal experience of teaching and learning, as either a student, mentor or parent, think about the different stages of evaluation you have come into contact with. You may have identified some of the following:

■ **Professional course evaluation**   Courses in nursing and midwifery have clear evaluation structures that enable them to ensure that they are meeting both the needs of the student and the outcomes set out for the course.

■ **Structures set up by government**    For example, the publication of league tables by the government to identify which schools are meeting the standards they have set. In higher education; the Quality Assurance Agency for Higher Education (QAA) is charged with reviewing the quality of higher education. Its purpose is to get best value from the investment made by the public by setting up clear mechanisms for quality assurance; to make the processes for evaluation open and transparent; and to encourage improvement by frequent re-evaluation of subjects being taught (Nicklin and Kenworthy 2000).

We all need to evaluate many aspects of our personal as well as our working lives. You might evaluate how well your coat was cleaned by the dry cleaners, or how effective you think your son's new teacher is; or you may evaluate the delivery of client care or the process of teaching and learning. The purpose of any evaluation process here is to improve upon outcomes, teaching processes or learning achievement, and ultimately to benefit patient/client care. We may also need to evaluate to ensure the cost-effectiveness of the delivery of learning. In some circumstances, an evaluation process that identifies poor learning or poor client care may mean that drastic measures need to be taken, such as stopping an education programme or withdrawing learners from a particular care environment. We may also need to submit a formal evaluation of teaching and learning in order to fulfil the requirements of specific educational programmes.

(The process of evaluating teaching and learning should identify whether or not the teaching methods used were appropriate, whether the strategy to deliver the programme fitted the situation, whether the assessment methods used were the best choice for the topic or outcomes being assessed and, indeed, whether the learning outcomes had been developed correctly.)

Evaluation may illustrate different aspects of what has been taught and what has been learned. It may demonstrate that the two do not match, and that failure to learn may result from the teaching process rather than the learning process. The process of evaluation provides everyone concerned with the information necessary to move forward.

## When is the best time to evaluate?

Evaluation is sometimes seen as the end of a process. In reality, it is part of a circular process to which there is no end, but where the results of evaluation lead back to the assessment – or reassessment – of a situation, for example patients'/clients' care needs, or a learner's needs in an educational programme.

However, it could be argued that when and how frequently to evaluate depends upon what and how much is being taught and learned, and, in practical terms, on the time available to teach and learn. For example, a nursing student may only be with you for a very short time, but his learning, while on placement, needs not only to be assessed but also evaluated. This could lead to repeated, rather superficial evaluation. On the other hand, if a learner's placement with you is for longer, or if the evaluation is for a permanent member of staff, the process might take much longer and be more individualised. If we look at the question of when to evaluate when using the Knowledge and Skills Framework (KSF), as described earlier, then we can see that evaluation is at the end of one cycle in a development review and the start of the next. Therefore the probable answer to 'when' to evaluate is, 'whenever necessary'!

## Where is the most appropriate place to evaluate?

Evaluation should take place wherever teaching and learning take place. Depending on your role, this might be in the practice setting, so you need to tailor your evaluation processes to reflect this. Remember that evaluation will also be undertaken by all the other people involved with the whole programme of learning, and your evaluation should contribute to the total picture – it is one piece in a jigsaw.

## What is it we need to evaluate?

There are two facets that need to be addressed in evaluation processes. The first covers the concrete, factual, physical components that can be identified in any teaching and/or learning situation and which are easily measurable. They can be linked to the learning outcomes or criteria pertinent to a programme.

In relation to knowledge and skills, there may be tight controls on what is evaluated; for example, in the National Vocational Qualification and Scottish Vocational Qualification (NVQ/SVQ) awards, the amount, complexity and level of skill and knowledge the learner must achieve before he can be said to be competent are clearly identified. Similar processes are seen in most programmes, and the standards that must be achieved and maintained are often specified; thus, it is easy to measure the extent to which they have been met. This evaluation approach measures output against input and is sometimes termed a **scientific evaluation** (Ellington et al. 1993).

Another area of evaluation relates to the systems and processes that support and contribute to the fixed components of the programme – in other words, the variables contained in any learning process. This is sometimes called **illuminative evaluation** (Ellington et al. 1993).

The **learning environment** is a vital component here. As you are probably most closely involved with the practice area, you will be very aware of how the climate can change – sometimes at a moment's notice, often dramatically – and how these changes can affect the results of an evaluation process carried out by learners. Just think for a moment about how the atmosphere changes when a senior staff member has an 'off day', or a clinical crisis, such as a cardiac arrest, occurs.

**ACTIVITY 5.2**   Think of two learners who spent the same length of time with you in your area, but who gave very different evaluations of their experiences. Why do you think their evaluations were different?

You may have listed your relationships with individual learners, or the progress made with them, and how this may have affected your 'input' and hence their 'output'. Although it would be ideal to suggest that all learners receive the same input from you it is unrealistic to expect this, because you, the learner and the environment, are not the same from day to day. An evaluation occurs at a particular moment in time and thus gives a snapshot of what happened at that time.

As with most learning processes there may be additional benefits felt and gained by some learners – spin-offs, such as increased confidence in their own ability and the improvement of their communication skills. These are all bonuses in any learning programme. The attitudes of learners, including their perceptions and opinions, may also be evaluated in this context, as may the attitudes of other staff involved with the support and teaching of learners. Most evaluation systems will incorporate a mixture of the scientific and illuminative components in order to give a broad and deep understanding of the processes involved and the results achieved.

## Who are we going to evaluate?

As this chapter is entitled 'Evaluating Learning and Teaching', it may be obvious that who is being evaluated is you, your learners and, to a lesser extent, the other people involved in the learning process. This also suggests that these people are the ones who undertake the process of evaluation, using methods detailed later in the chapter.

## HOW TO EVALUATE TEACHING

A number of methods can be used to evaluate learning and teaching, and, as you will find out, most can be used for both purposes. However, the aim of this section is to explore the evaluation of teaching. These are aspects of evaluation that can help you in this process.

## Self-evaluation

Self-evaluation can help you to identify personal progress, to clarify what is still to be learned, and to recognise how past learning can be incorporated into current practices (Burnard 1988).

If, in your evaluation, you identify that some students have failed to learn, then something has gone wrong. It may be that the objectives, learning outcomes or components of the learning contract were unrealistic and did not fit the overall programme aims; or it may be that the methods used to deliver those outcomes were inappropriate to the learning style of the individual student.

Whatever has gone wrong, you need to evaluate your methods and processes in order to identify the problem and correct it. If you do not evaluate yourself, there is a tendency to carry on as usual. The process of self-evaluation allows you to reflect and prepare yourself for future learning.

In your professional role you may have a great deal of personal autonomy, together with personal and professional accountability. The autonomy allows you, as an individual, to determine how you practise, in parameters set by, for example, your employer, your linked educational institution and the Nursing and Midwifery Council (NMC). This autonomy is a privilege and enables you to develop as an independent practitioner, teacher, mentor and assessor in your practice environment, so you need to be rigorous and active in maintaining and developing your standards in these areas (Reece and Walker 1997). Because of this, you will be expected to monitor your own standards and to review and evaluate your own delivery, whether this relates to patient/client care or to teaching and assessing learners. This evaluation will enable you to undertake a SWOT analysis:

S = Strengths
W = Weaknesses
O = Opportunities
T = Threats.

---

**ACTIVITY 5.3**   Undertake a SWOT analysis in relation to your role as a teacher. Your responses might be:

- Strengths – confidence, enthusiasm, experience
- Weaknesses – time, other competing commitments
- Opportunities – working environment, teaching and/or assessor programme
- Threats – work demands, other staff, other learners.

---

You are accountable to your learners to offer them the best opportunities to learn and progress.

One way to evaluate yourself is through a self-evaluation (or reflective) diary, and through the development of a personal professional portfolio (see Chapter 4). According to Andrews (1996), reflecting on action has two properties in common with evaluation: that is, both are purposeful and active processes. You are involved with updating and expanding your professional development in response to the NMC's post-registration education and practice (PREP) requirements. It would seem logical to use your development as a teacher and assessor in your practice environment to fulfil some of these requirements, and a reflective diary, which not only details the processes you have gone through, but also shows how you have learned from these situations and improved your skills, will go some way towards meeting the NMC's requirements. This reflection will also fit your requirements in respect of Dimension 2 of the KSF, namely Personal and People Development, and will give you evidence for your own personal development plan.

In *The PREP Handbook* (NMC 2002) it is suggested that you may wish to work through the following stages when planning your professional portfolio:

1.  Review your competence. What are your strengths, areas that you need to develop, and areas for further personal development?

2.  Set your learning objectives. What do you want to achieve?

3.  Develop an action plan. What learning activities will help you to meet your needs?

4.  Implement the action plan. Discuss your plan with your manager, link tutor or other relevant personnel.

5.  Evaluate what happened. Once you have implemented the action plan, you can think about what happened and what you have learned.

6.  Record your study time and learning outcomes. Accurately record all your learning activities.

All of these areas can be addressed in such a way as to encompass your teaching and assessing roles, and the format should enable you to evaluate your techniques, your individual style and your development in relation to these skills, while at the same time meeting your PREP requirements.

Maintaining a personal professional portfolio enables you to keep a record of your professional development, whether in clinical practice, teaching or assessing. However, it is more than a record of achievement and should be based upon a regular process of reflection and, by implication, evaluation. The benefits of this process are numerous and include the development of analytical skills that you will be able to apply, not only to your own personal and professional growth, but also to the growth of others. Furthermore, such skills help you to assess your current standards of practice and to demonstrate experiential learning, all of which may allow you to obtain credit towards further qualifications.

In programmes that enable you to develop your teaching and assessing skills, this process of reflection can help you to evaluate yourself. Others will also assess you and evaluate your learning, as you will be observed by the tutors involved with course delivery, and their observation of your sessions will be documented.

In this section you have looked at evaluating your own teaching and learning, but you need to examine other ways of evaluating your teaching and methods of assessing learning in your clinical environment. Some of these methods can, of course, be used to evaluate patient/client care, but in your role as teacher and assessor you need to evaluate whether your nursing students, health care assistants (HCAs), newly qualified staff and those staff you are supporting in developing their own KSF, have benefited from their experiences and exposure to learning opportunities in your clinical environment.

## Gaining feedback

Evaluative feedback can be gained from a number of sources, via a wide range of methods. In many cases a variety of evaluation techniques are used in order to gain an overall view of the effectiveness of learning and teaching. Your evaluation processes will probably relate to a self-contained unit of learning, which will be specific to your clinical environment and the learners in it.

The outcome of evaluation should, therefore, aim to identify and demonstrate the appropriateness of:

- Teaching methods
- The structure adopted
- The implementation strategy
- Assessment methods
- The learning objectives.

The methods that can be used to ascertain these are:

- Checklists
- Interviews
- Questionnaires

- Results from learner assessment
- Feedback from other staff.

Use of any of the methods listed above is an individual choice, but it is your responsibility to select the methods best suited to your needs. There is no single correct way to undertake evaluation. The methods selected may differ according to whether you are evaluating the scientific component of a programme or session, evaluating the additional benefits through an illuminative approach, or attempting to evaluate both.

## CHECKLISTS

Checklists can be used to start the self-evaluation process. A checklist should be seen as an aide-mémoire to the whole process of evaluation.

Most people are relatively familiar with a checklist approach. Think, for example, of when you go shopping and make a list; or when you prepare to undertake a clinical procedure and how you mentally (or physically) tick off the points as you go along. For example, when preparing to undertake an aseptic technique, your list might look like this:

- Trolley, appropriately prepared
- Dressing pack
- Cleansing solution
- Strapping
- Extra swabs/forceps
- Wound swab (just in case!)

However, when you prepare to undertake a teaching session your list may include:

- Room booked
- Learners aware of session, topic, time and place
- Teaching aids available
- Learning objectives prepared
- Audiovisual aids prepared
- Overall session prepared
- Self prepared!

This information can be gathered before you start a session and fed into the whole evaluative process at the end. The next stage is to deliver the teaching session in question. During this session you will be able to ascertain whether or not it is going well – intrinsic feedback can be gained from your activities, that is, you have an immediate idea of how you are performing, using such indicators as the learners' attention and the expression on their faces. This immediate feedback is important, as it might enable you to alter your presentation 'on the hoof', if possible, or to take this information into account when evaluating the whole session in order to make alterations for next time.

## INTERVIEWS

A more formal method that you can use to evaluate your teaching is to question the group or individuals from the group. For this to be useful you need to ask specific and objective questions that can be answered by the individuals involved. It may be very difficult for learners to answer questions that need a personal response, especially about you, when they know that they will be working with you again and that you will be assessing their practice. It is best, therefore, if learners' evaluations concentrate on the teaching and learning process rather than on the teacher's competence (Ward-Griffin and Brown 1992). However, a structured interview may enable you to address some items in greater depth than questionnaires permit, and subsequent questions may develop because of responses to previous questions.

Interviews can be difficult to control at times, and it is all too easy to digress. In order to elicit the information required, it is advisable to prepare your questions in advance and set yourself a time limit for the interview. You will obviously need to record the outcomes of the interview; this could be done using an audiotape, with the learners' permission, or by making notes during the activity. However, it is difficult to make notes when someone is talking: think back to the time you spent in a classroom, trying to make notes, and listen and understand what was being said, all at the same time. Remember that you must be able to interpret the information later, when the learner is not there to explain what he said or why, so make sure your notes are readable and comprehensive, and that you can understand them. Adequate preparation beforehand will greatly reduce any problems later.

## QUESTIONNAIRES

It may be more appropriate to devise a questionnaire to distribute to the group, especially where the content and process is the same and will be repeated with different individuals – by using this method you may be able to cover more aspects. Your questionnaire can be completed anonymously and be handed in for analysis and collation. The content must obviously apply to the topic and session concerned, but can draw on both the scientific and the illuminative approaches.

Ideally, you should use both open questions, which will need a written and therefore an individual response, and closed questions, which will require only a tick. Closed questions are easier to answer and easier to collate. By using questionnaires as an evaluation method you are undertaking research into your teaching, and by using both open and closed questions you are aiming to collect both qualitative and quantitative data.

The key to any questionnaire lies in its response rate (that is, the number of people who actually complete it as a percentage of those to whom it was given). A poor response rate will not give you a fair picture, so one way of aiming for a good response rate is to keep the questionnaire simple and answerable.

**ACTIVITY 5.4**   Consider any questionnaires that you might have completed in the past. What made some easy to complete? What made others difficult? Your responses to the first question might include:

- The length of the questionnaire
- The layout
- The language used;

and to the second question, your responses might be:

- Too long
- Too crowded
- Confusing/ambiguous language.

Ideally a questionnaire should take no longer than 4 or 5 minutes to complete, and telling respondents where to return the questionnaires is vital or you will not get them back.

You will need to decide when to distribute your questionnaire – either at the beginning or the end of your session. Whichever you choose, you need a speedy return of the completed forms, soon after the end of the session, in order to obtain an accurate response from your learners before failing memory or discussion with others can distort or alter the accuracy of their responses.

Once you have collected your completed questionnaires, you will need to collate and analyse the information obtained. You will probably be collecting both qualitative and quantitative data.

Once you have done this you may need to alter your session according to the results, repeat the session in its amended version, and then re-evaluate it.

Remember that the process of evaluation and the development and redevelopment of your teaching should be an ongoing and cyclical process.

# HOW TO EVALUATE LEARNING

Much of this topic is covered in the section on self-evaluation, as this relates to all learners, whatever their role or course. Your learners should be encouraged to undertake a process of self-evaluation related to both theory and practice. Many of them will also be encouraged and expected to produce a reflective diary. It is almost impossible to evaluate teaching without evaluating what learning has taken place, so that you can apply all of the topics discussed in the previous section when you evaluate learning.

It can be seen that many of the topics already covered in this chapter refer to all learners in your clinical environment. However, there are some methods of evaluation that focus primarily on evaluating teaching.

Probably the most obvious way for you to evaluate the learning that has taken place is through the assessment of learners in your workplace. Remember that assessment normally takes place before evaluation, but the results of evaluation feed into the next cycle of the planning and implementation of your teaching, which leads to the assessment of the next group of learners, and so on. Now you need to collect the information gathered through assessment and feed it into evaluation. Sound evaluation does not simply rely on information from one source but uses as much information as possible from every source, method and process available.

| **ACTIVITY 5.5** | Think through your own experiences, both as a teacher and as a learner, and list the issues that demonstrate success in learning. Your list might include: |
|---|---|

- Motivated learners
- A motivated teacher with the appropriate knowledge and skills to teach the topic
- An environment conducive to learning
- Clearly defined and achievable learning objectives, which may be set out in a learning contract and agreement
- A sound link between the practice setting and the educational establishment (if appropriate)
- Support for both learners and teachers/assessors
- The use of appropriate methods of assessment that give the information needed for evaluation
- Time!

If it is shown that learning has not taken place evaluation should identify where any problem lies, and it can therefore give you some information on how to improve this for the next time.

## Peer evaluation

One area that applies to the evaluation of both teaching and learning is peer evaluation. In the evaluation of learning, Burnard (1988) suggests that peer evaluation can follow immediately from the process of self-evaluation, by sharing your self-evaluation in a small group and inviting group members to comment and offer feedback. This process has the advantage of developing self-awareness and can be used when evaluating a module of learning.

There are disadvantages to this process, inasmuch as it can be difficult to confront your own failings, but to have your peers confirm these findings, even constructively, can be both disheartening and destructive. In order for peer evaluation to be considered worthwhile, the group involved should be cohesive and supportive, with self-confident members who are also confident in their peers. The group facilitator (which may be you as the teacher) must be able to handle the session effectively, in order to achieve a positive and constructive outcome.

## Evaluating the effectiveness of your teaching

So far we have looked at evaluation in relation to assessment and student feedback. This section will look specifically at the different evaluation methods you may wish to adopt before, during and after your teaching session.

When evaluating a teaching session, the key questions for resolution are, what exactly are you going to evaluate and, probably more importantly, why? This is crucial, as it will ultimately determine the strategy you adopt.

**ACTIVITY 5.6**   Make a list of the benefits you feel can be gained for both students and teachers by evaluating your teaching methods as opposed to what has been learned.

Under the 'student' heading you may have included aspects such as the 'feelgood factor'. The fact that the teacher is openly evaluating the effectiveness of her teaching often acts as a motivator, also providing the student with a clear picture of what she has learned.

For the teacher, evaluation provides an excellent framework for improving the session. For example, you may have incorporated role-play into your session and, following evaluation, now feel that a discussion group would have been more appropriate. Kiger (1995, p. 221) states that 'evaluation is an inevitable and essential part of the teaching–learning process'.

**ACTIVITY 5.7**   What do you think Kiger meant by the above statement? What does the statement mean to you? Why it is both inevitable and essential?

You may have included issues such as the students' opinion of the value of the teaching session, or whether the teacher felt that she had explained the subject in a way that was easily understood. Kiger (1995) terms this 'informal evaluation' and suggests that this takes place regardless of any strategic plan.

Abbatt and McMahon (1993) identify three aspects that can be effectively evaluated by the teacher: the plan, the process and the product.

## EVALUATING THE TEACHING PLAN

This involves all of the preparation undertaken by the teacher prior to the teaching taking place. This may be a 'one-off' teaching session, in either the practice or the college environment, or a full course or module. It may appear almost contradictory to talk about evaluating a teaching session before it has begun, but there are many aspects of teaching that will greatly increase the likelihood of the content of the session or course being appropriate. To this end, there are some fundamental questions that you can ask once you have amassed your teaching material and clearly written your plan.

- Have you considered and included any instructions you have been given? For example, the session may be one of a sequence. If so, does your preparation follow on logically from the previous session and lead logically on to the next?

- Can you fulfil the objectives you have set for yourself with the content of the session?

- Will you be able to complete the session in the time you have been allocated?

- Is your teaching pitched at the right level for the group or student you are about to teach? For example, you would expect a third-year student to have a greater understanding of how to care for an unconscious patient than one in her first year.

- How confident are you with the teaching methods you will use? From previous chapters, it is clear that using a variety of teaching methods both enhances the learning process and leads to a much more enjoyable learning experience.

- Are your objectives sufficiently clear to ensure that the student understands what is to be gained from the session?

**ACTIVITY 5.8**    Take some time to think about how you could find out if you have fulfilled your
objectives.
   The most straightforward way is probably to ask the students. For example,
you can pose a question directly relating to the objective and hope for an appropriate response. It is crucial to acknowledge, however, that it may only tell you
that one student (or however many answer the question correctly) has an understanding, but it does not tell you about the whole class. Generally, it is valuable to
use the first 5–10 minutes of any teaching session discussing with the students
what they can expect to gain from it.

## EVALUATING THE TEACHING PROCESS

Abbatt and McMahon (1993) argue that evaluation of the process of teaching centres largely on observation and discussion. Before these aspects are
developed in relation to your teaching plan, however, it may be useful to
identify what is actually meant by the process of teaching. A straightforward definition of process (*Concise Oxford Dictionary* 1983) is the 'state of
going on or being carried on' – this type of evaluation can take place during the time the subject material is being delivered.

A great deal of information can be gained by observation. This may be
by the teacher delivering the session or by other teachers, when it is known
as peer review – discussed earlier in this chapter.

### Use of checklists/questionnaires in evaluation

A checklist is useful to enable you to identify aspects of your teaching that
you could improve on, and it is particularly valuable when used at the same
time as students' written evaluations.

There are many tools available to assist you in this, all of which identify
five or six key areas for evaluation:

1. **The teacher's presentation of the subject material**    This involves the
   practical aspects of subject delivery, for example:
   - Could the teacher be heard?
   - Did the teaching follow a logical progression?
   - Was the teaching delivered in words that the students understood?
   - Were the visual aids used in the support of teaching clear and
     appropriate?

2. **The teacher's approach to the students**    This includes questions such as:
   - Was the teacher enthusiastic about the subject?
   - Was the teacher able to establish a rapport with the students?

- Was the teacher able to recognise the need for student participation?
- Did the teacher respond sensitively to the students?

3. **Student understanding and participation**
   - Were the students encouraged effectively to become involved in the teaching session?
   - Was the learning related to the students' previous experience?
   - Was student interest maintained throughout the session?
   - Was the students' level of knowledge elicited at the start, in order to build on this?

4. **Meeting objectives**
   - Were the objectives for the session discussed with the students?
   - Were the objectives appropriate?
   - Were the objectives specific and unambiguous?
   - Were the objectives shared with the students?

5. **The teaching and learning environment**
   - Was the general environment conducive to learning, for example not too hot, too cold or too small?
   - Were surrounding noise levels acceptable?
   - Were the furnishings and teaching aids of an acceptable standard?

6. **Feedback**
   - Were students given immediate, appropriate and unambiguous feedback on the points they raised during the session?
   - Were students advised on how they could improve their understanding and find our more information?

Using the list above as a framework you should be able to develop your own evaluation tool, which can then be adapted to meet any teaching situation, either in the classroom or the practice setting, and with individuals or groups.

## EVALUATING THE TEACHING PRODUCT

This type of evaluation tends to be more relevant to a course or module, as it involves more formal assessment and examination processes. For example, a high pass rate at examination is a reasonably good indicator that the product is satisfactory and that the criteria laid down for it are being met. Whatever the type of evaluation used, one aspect is fundamental to them all – that is, the need to act on the findings in order to improve the ways in which we teach.

# EVALUATING AND ASSESSING COMPETENCE

Having looked at how you can ensure that students get the most from your teaching, this part of the chapter provides some practical advice on how you can assess their competence in practice and is closely tied into your role as mentor, either formally or informally, or as a formal assessor through the vocational qualifications (VQ) framework.

## The value of learning in and from practice

The government's modernisation agenda for the NHS has placed a great deal of emphasis on learning in and from practice. The workplace is viewed as a very rich place to learn, not only in and between different health care professions, but also for all workers with a health care role. This, however, places a heavy responsibility on the workforce, charged both with supporting learning in practice and with the responsibility for ensuring their competence at the level at which they are required to work.

| ACTIVITY 5.9 | Make a list of the benefits that you feel could be gained from both learning and supporting students in the workplace. |
|---|---|

You will probably have identified some of the following:

- Potential cost benefits for both the individual and the organisation. It is particularly helpful to the employer as there are no costs involved in replacing essential staff while they undertake study away from the work environment

- You are able to observe the students in action

- You are able to demonstrate and repeat procedures as required

- You are potentially able to discuss issues as they arise

- You are able, to some extent, to control the learning environment. For example, you are able to assess whether you feel it appropriate that the student be involved in difficult or challenging situations with patients or clients.

## What is competence and why do we need to measure it?

A straightforward definition of competence is the ability to undertake a certain task or procedure, although in the provision of health care it is necessary for us to widen this to include issues such as safety and level. For example, it is not enough, in terms of patient safety, simply to be able to inject a substance such as insulin: it is also important to be able to do it safely. As a result, the United Kingdom Central Council (UKCC 1999), then nursing's regulatory body, defined competence as 'the skills and ability to practise safely and effectively without the need for direct supervision'. (Note that in 2002 the UKCC was replaced by the Nursing and Midwifery Council) But there is more to it than that: in the plethora of available defin-itions, reference is made not only to skills that are observable but also to unobservable attributes, including the rather subjective issue of attitudes (Benner 1984).

As we can see from the above, the term competence can have a variety of definitions, and it is perhaps easier to consider a consolidated definition of competence as suggested by Storey et al. (2002), which is:

> Competence is the knowledge, skills, abilities and behaviours that a practitioner needs to perform their work to a professional standard, and is a key lever for achieving results that will enable the organisation to achieve its health care objectives.

There are many ways in which to monitor whether these have been achieved.

---

**ACTIVITY 5.10**   How could you be confident that your student is competent in a specific task? Make a list of how you would know.

---

Your answers may have included some of the following:

- Watch him or her so that you can assure yourself that the student is doing the task correctly.

- Ask them questions to ascertain their level of understanding.

- Ask someone with a sound knowledge of the student to provide a written report.

- Scrutinise their written work.

- Look at materials they have produced, e.g. a portfolio.

In recent years, nurses involved in the assessment of practice have been called mentors, assessors or both; for the purposes of VQ assessment (discussed later) the term assessor is used. The term mentor is used to denote the role of the nurse, midwife or health visitor who facilitates learning and supervises and assesses students in the practice setting (ENB/DoH 2001, p. 9). In order to minimise confusion in this chapter, the terms mentor and assessor are used interchangeably.

# ASSESSING COMPETENCE PRE- AND POST-REGISTRATION

## Mentor responsibilities

The key responsibilities of mentors have been clearly identified by the Royal College of Nursing (2002). Mentors need to:

- Contribute to a supportive learning environment and quality learning outcomes for students
- Be approachable and supportive and have knowledge of how students learn best
- Have knowledge and information about the student's programme of study and practice assessment tools in use throughout the UK
- Be willing to share their knowledge of patient/client care
- Identify specific learning opportunities that are available in the placement area
- Ensure that the learning experience is a planned process
- Ensure that time is identified for initial interviews with students, in order to assess learning needs
- Develop a learning contract or logs as appropriate
- Identify with students their 'core competencies and outcomes to be achieved' by the end of the placement
- Make time to observe students undertaking new skills for the first time and also when practising newly learned skills
- Encourage the application of enquiry-based learning and problem solving to situations rather than just giving factual information
- Build into the learning experiences opportunities to experience the skills and knowledge of other specialist practitioners
- Build into the daily routine adequate break times to enable students to enjoy the practice learning experience

- Offer encouragement to students to work in partnership with the multiprofessional team in order to provide holistic care

- Provide time for reflection, feedback and monitoring of students' progress

- Ensure that students have constructive positive feedback with suggestions for how they can make further improvement to promote progress

- Seek evaluative feedback from students at the end of their practice placement

- Be willing to take pride in sharing the students' journey towards becoming a registered nurse or midwife.

## Mentorship preparation

The UKCC (now the NMC in 2002) identified advisory standards for mentors and mentorship – and the importance of eight key areas to the mentorship process:

1. Communication and working relationships, including:
   - The development of effective relationships based on mutual trust and respect
   - An understanding of how students integrate into practice settings and assisting with this process
   - The provision of ongoing constructive support for students

2. Facilitation of learning in order to:
   - Demonstrate sufficient knowledge of the students' programme to identify current learning needs
   - Demonstrate strategies that will assist with the integration of learning from practice and education settings
   - Create and develop opportunities for students to identify and undertake experiences to meet their learning needs

3. Assessment in order to:
   - Demonstrate effective relationships with patients and clients
   - Contribute to the development of an environment in which effective practice is fostered, implemented evaluated and disseminated
   - Assess and manage clinical developments to ensure safe and effective care

4.  Role modelling in order to:
    - Demonstrate effective relationships with patients and clients
    - Contribute to the development of an environment in which effective practice is fostered, implemented evaluated and disseminated
    - Assess and manage clinical developments to ensure safe and effective care

5.  Creating an environment for learning in order to:
    - Ensure effective learning experiences and the opportunity to achieve learning outcomes for students by contributing to the development and maintenance of a learning environment
    - Implement strategics for quality assurance and quality audit

6.  Improving practice in order to:
    - Contribute to the creation of an environment in which change can be initiated and supported

7.  A knowledge-base in order to:
    - Identify apply and disseminate research findings within the area of practice

8.  Course development that:
    - Contributes to the development and or/review of courses.

Nurses and midwives who take on the role of mentor must have current registration with the NMC. They will have completed at least 12 months' full-time experience (or equivalent part time). Mentors will require preparation for and support in their role. This should include access to a lecturer and/or practice educator as well as support from their line manager (NMC 2000, p. 11).

## ASSESSING COMPETENCE:  THE NVQ/SVQ FRAMEWORK

This part of the chapter covers the concepts, uses and applications of NVQs and SVQs as a competence framework used in the health care workplace, with particular reference to those awards devised for the assessment of competence in care delivery.

As identified in Chapter 2, NVQs and SVQs have been developed at five levels. At present, NVQs and SVQs in Care are at levels 2, 3 and 4, with the greatest uptake of these awards currently being at level 2. This is followed by level 3, where numbers are increasing, and then at level 4, where uptake in the health care sector is still relatively low, though growing quite rapidly in the social care sector, which includes staff in nursing homes. However, there are a number of other NVQs and SVQs that are used in health care settings, for example:

- HCAs, registered nurses and midwives may undertake Management awards at levels 3, 4 and 5
- HCAs, registered nurses and midwives may use the National Occupational Standards (NOS) in Health Promotion
- Assessors across and in a variety of disciplines, including professional and non-professional staff, working towards and achieving the NVQ/SVQ assessor and verifier awards (A and V units) which are discrete, standalone NOS from larger awards in the Training and Development suite of awards
- Managers, including nurses, in residential and nursing homes for example, will work towards, and achieve, the Residential Managers (Adult) award at level 4.

The care awards at levels 2, 3 and 4 cover a vast range of staff, from HCAs employed in residential and nursing homes and acute care environments, to HCAs employed in primary care trusts (PCT) working with district nurses, and midwives and in GP practices. The current NVQs and SVQs in care, namely:

- Care level 2
- Blood donor support level 2
- Operating department support level 2
- Care level 3
- Promoting independence level 3
- Dialysis support level 3
- Diagnostic and therapeutic support level 3

are undergoing a review, which will be completed by the summer of 2004.

## QCA as a regulatory body

The body responsible for NVQs in England, Wales and Northern Ireland is the Qualifications and Curriculum Authority (QCA). In Scotland this role is undertaken by the Scottish Qualifications Authority (SQA). At the heart of QCA's work is the establishment of a coherent national framework of qualifications, of which NVQs are just one strand, and which also includes General Certificates of Secondary Education (GCSE), 'A' levels and Vocational 'A' levels (previously GNVQ), Higher National Certificates (HNC) and Higher National Diplomas (HND). In this chapter the emphasis is on NVQs/SVQs, which 'set the seal on standards of performance established for specific occupations'. NVQs are work-based and are designed to 'provide open access to assessment and facilitate lifelong learning for people in employment' (QCA 1997a). The role of QCA is to:

- Accredit qualifications put forward by awarding bodies, if they meet the published criteria
- Ensure the quality of the overall qualification system through working with awarding bodies
- Monitor the performance and effectiveness of the awarding bodies through quality audits.

There are seven stages in the development of an NVQ:

- The establishment of the standard-setting body, e.g. the Sector Skills Council (SSC), namely Skills for Health, established in 2003
- The SSC draws up the standards of competence that will form the NVQ, ensuring appropriate and adequate consultation with employers
- Awarding bodies, e.g. City and Guilds, Edexcel and SQA, work with the SSC to develop assessment and quality assurance arrangements in order to ensure that the proposed standards can be delivered as a qualification
- The QCA considers the proposals against their criteria
- Contracts are agreed with QCA and awarding bodies for the NVQ to be made available to the public and to be entered on to the NVQ database
- Accreditation is given for a period of time – no longer than 5 years – and during this time QCA monitors the actions of the awarding body in respect of the approved NVQ
- The SSC continually reviews the standards and the NVQ structure to ensure it remains up to date and fit for purpose.

At the end of the agreed period awarding bodies make a submission to QCA for reaccreditation of the NVQ and the cycle starts again.

## Awarding bodies

These are the organisations approved by the QCA to award qualifications in England, Wales and Northern Ireland. SQA fulfils this regulatory function and also the function of awarding body in Scotland. Many NVQ/SVQs apply to and are used in health and social care environments, and as noted earlier, the most common are the suite of Care awards, Management awards and Training and Development awards. The role of the awarding bodies is to:

- Ensure the quality and consistency of assessment for qualifications nationally
- Produce guidance for approved centres to offer the awards
- Appoint, support and develop external verifiers, allocate them to approved centres and monitor their work
- Approve and monitor centres against the approved centre criteria
- Collect information from approved centres to inform national decisions about qualification delivery
- Provide information to QCA.

There are a number of awarding bodies offering NVQ/SVQs, but in the care framework these are the City and Guilds of London Institute – the care section in this body being known as City and Guilds Affinity – and a partnership between BTEC and the Institute for Health Care Delivery known as Edexcel. These bodies also function in Scotland, as does the SQA in its role of awarding body.

## Approved assessment centres

These are organisations approved by awarding bodies to offer, assess, verify and award qualifications. Their role is to:

- Manage assessment and verification on a day-to-day basis
- Have effective assessment practices and internal verification procedures
- Meet awarding body requirements for qualification delivery
- Have sufficient competent assessors and internal verifiers with enough time and authority to carry out their roles effectively.

Approved centres come in many guises in the health care sector, ranging from an individual NHS Trust – often a Training and Development

Department – to a consortium of nursing homes working together in partnership to offer awards, through to an independent training agency offering awards across a vast spectrum of qualifications. Whatever the composition of the approved centre, they all have to meet the criteria stated above, although they will meet them in different ways and through different processes. Awarding bodies set criteria by which they evaluate the applications for centre approval and carry out ongoing monitoring of centres through their external verifier processes. The criteria are devised in order to ensure that a centre is able to:

- Deliver the assessment process

- Ensure the quality of assessment.

Subsequently the criteria:

- Help to ensure consistency in centre approval and monitoring across qualifications and awarding bodies

- Specify the systems, resources and quality assurance arrangements that a centre needs to establish and maintain

- Act as performance indicators against which a centre's performance can be evaluated and monitored

- Establish a framework and reporting structure for discussions after approval between the centre and QCA quality audit staff (QCA 1997b).

You may be wondering at this point why you need to have all of the above information! The answer is that this information demonstrates the robust framework and audit processes that are involved before any HCAs or other health care staff can undertake such awards and obtain these qualifications.

## Different supporting roles

So, where do you fit in this process? You may be undertaking a number of roles in supporting staff through NVQ/SVQs; these may be as an assessor, teacher, course coordinator or internal verifier. It is worth noting here that NVQ/SVQs are not prescribed taught programmes, demanding attendance at lectures and seminars, though these may be an agreed part of the delivery from your workplace perspective. Rather, NVQ/SVQs are about the individual undertaking the award – let us call them the candidate – demonstrating to their assessor that, through a variety of methods, they have acquired the correct knowledge and can perform skills to an acceptable standard: in other words, they have acquired and demonstrated competence. Much of your work with NVQ/SVQ candidates will entail teaching and assessing. It is very difficult to separate the two concepts, so it is probably appropriate here to look at the format of NVQ/SVQ awards so that you can have the full picture of the processes and where you fit in them.

## NVQ/SVQ structure

NVQs and SVQs are ultimately qualifications made up of a number of units of competence. These units of competence are the building bricks of the structure, but can also be used as standalone tools by which to assess competence in a selected role, using a nationally accredited tool with a rigorous audited infrastructure. This is worth remembering, as, for example, 9 or 12 units cannot possibly encompass the entire role of an HCA. Rather, these units cover the areas where it is considered vital that rigorous assessment of knowledge and practice is best focused, in order to achieve the best outcomes in relation to care delivery.

**ACTIVITY 5.11**    Think about an HCA in your practice area. List the skills and roles she performs on a daily basis. Match these to the NVQ/SVQ award structure and identify any gaps.

You may have listed areas such as direct patient care, e.g. hygiene needs, toileting needs, mobility needs, nutritional needs, patient handling, care of people who are dying, looking after surgical wounds, caring for patients with incontinence, record keeping, communication, maintaining stock, taking baseline observations such as blood pressure, obtaining venous and/or capillary blood samples, etc.

There are 14 separate skills listed here, already well over the 12 units for a level 3 award, and probably still not covering the whole of the HCA's role. NVQs and SVQs have been developed as 'pick and mix' awards, although there may be restrictions in the 'pick and mix' options. There are mandatory core units, including health and safety and equality, which all HCAs undertaking both levels 2 and 3 must achieve. Other units are based upon their award level and their role in the care team. It is worth reminding yourself here of the definitions of the levels of NVQ/SVQ contained in Chapter 2.

You might find that your HCA may have undertaken a level 2 award but is really working in the definition of level 3. If this process is reversed

**ACTIVITY 5.12**    Reread the definitions of NVQ/SVQ in Chapter 2, and then think of an HCA in your area and match her to one level in the definitions.

you may need to ask if that HCA is working to her appropriate capacity and competence. Movement from level 2 to level 3 is *not* automatic, but can only be undertaken if the HCA's role and autonomy are extended, possibly through promotion, or in order to gain promotion. This links with the KSF detailed in Chapter 4. It is also not essential that HCAs have undertaken a level 2 award before they work towards a level 3: the level should have been chosen for compatibility with their role.

## Choice of units

You may now be asking who chooses the units that a particular individual will need to do in order to achieve a qualification. The best answer is to suggest a partnership approach here, which marries the needs of the area with the needs of the individual. You may have a number of HCAs in your area working towards these awards. If so, it is not necessary that they all undertake the same units. It may be possible – and indeed beneficial – for individuals working in a particular practice area to develop a skill mix in the HCA staff group, giving the best possible establishment of care-givers. Remember that the units chosen must fit the individual's role, as day-to-day working practices will form the basis of assessment. It is no good the HCA wanting to undertake a unit that involves caring for babies when she works on a ward caring for mentally frail older people. When the appropriate level and unit choices have been made, then the HCA will be registered for that award with the relevant body, through the assessment centre.

The units of competence are further broken down into elements, which are subsections of units, and these elements are then broken down into performance criteria (PC). These criteria give fine detail to the overall title of the element, and the elements give detail to the main subject of the unit. In reality, the PC can be seen as the 'doing' component of units of competence, and supporting them, in the whole unit structure, is a section containing knowledge evidence – the 'knowing' part of the unit. In effect, when the PC and the knowledge evidence are put together and taught and assessed so that competence is demonstrated, the candidate can be seen to have linked theory (knowledge) to practice. It is your role to make sure this link has been firmly made. So, overall, an NVQ/SVQ Unit can be illustrated as in Figure 5.1.

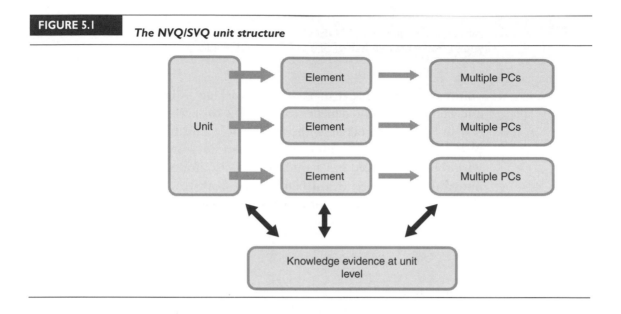

**FIGURE 5.1**    *The NVQ/SVQ unit structure*

## TEACHING AND ASSESSING – GETTING STARTED

As with most many other teaching and assessment processes, including those related to nursing students, with which you will be involved, you need to start by talking with your candidate and establishing a route through the award. This means establishing their current competence, including knowledge and skills, and matching those with the award and units to be undertaken. You may be teaching and assessing an HCA with whom you have worked for some considerable time, in which case some tact and diplomacy may be needed, especially if the award has become mandatory rather than optional in your area. Unlike nursing students, who move through a variety of care environments throughout their programme, HCAs tend to undertake their awards in their permanent area of employment. Equally, they may be new staff, in which case it is potentially easier to establish a framework for action.

Your HCA may feel very confident in his or her skills and may resent any formal assessment. This has to be done, but please use common sense when assessing someone you have worked alongside repeatedly. If there are problems with competence they should have been remedied when identified, not now! It is perfectly acceptable to shorten the assessment process in areas where you, as the assessor and teacher, are quite confident with the individual's performance.

Next, after establishing this baseline with your candidate, is to decide which units you will concentrate on first. In reality this is quite difficult, as care is delivered holistically, but there is nothing to stop you teaching and assessing in this manner. Indeed, City and Guilds, as one of the awarding bodies, currently recommends holistic assessment as best practice for NVQ/SVQs.

To illustrate this, consider the day-to-day activities of an HCA in a nursing home caring for frail elderly people. Without doubt, her role on a morning shift will include caring for the hygiene, elimination, nutritional and mobility needs of her clients; at the same time she will need to communicate with clients, other staff and visitors, and treat everyone equally. In NVQ/SVQ terms this work crosses over at least six units of competence. So, where do you start? My advice is: if you are newly involved with NVQ/SVQs, then choose one unit that you and your candidate already feel comfortable with and use this as your starting point. When working through this unit refer constantly to other areas of competence and their respective units, and make notes for reference for when you formally begin to work with those units. In this way you will move through the award with your candidate, but at the same time get to know other parts of the award, ready to go through the process again with your next candidate! If you are experienced with NVQ/SVQs then you should be able to use a holistic approach to working with your candidate. Identify a number of units that you will work on simultaneously, and plan the work to be undertaken on these, with and by your candidate. A cautionary note is needed here, as, on the whole candidates like the notion of finishing a complete unit and then moving on to the next, ticking units off as they near completion. Your candidate may feel he or she is not progressing well with a more integrated approach, but reassurance of success and eventual completion of six units in one go usually restores their confidence.

# Route planning

In planning the route through the award you will identify areas of work your candidate will need to undertake in order to demonstrate competence. In effect, these will form methods of assessment and will include some teaching on your part, either to individuals or to groups of candidates. So, you might choose to ask your candidate to write a care study of a client they are caring for, covering the specific unit(s) she is working on. This may, for example, cover the management of continence, and therefore demand a sound knowledge of the safe disposal of body waste and issues related to the prevention of infection and cross-infection. This knowledge-base may be quite detailed and it might be more effective and efficient for you to teach your HCA the necessary underpinning knowledge on a one-to-one basis. Her completed care study should then demonstrate her understanding, and your assessment of her skills and care delivery in this area. It should confirm to you that your HCA is applying her knowledge to practice.

Alternatively, you may use a seminar approach to cover salient points about the Health and Safety at Work Act and its application in the health care workplace, and follow this up with a quiz or a multiple-choice test. So, having decided on the path through – and your input to – the NVQ/SVQ process you and your candidate will devise a learning contract or assessment plan so that the candidate knows exactly what is expected and any target dates involved. In theory, NVQs and SVQs have no prescribed timescales attached to them, but it is becoming increasingly common for employers to set target dates, and therefore you will need to set short- and longer-term goals in order to meet these. For example, for a level 2 candidate you may set an overall timescale of 1 year, aiming at completion of one unit per month, which, when accounting for holidays etc., should be a realistic target. There is, however, nothing to stop you and your candidate working at a faster pace.

Let us recap here and look at the process so far. You need to:

1. Identify which level of award your candidate is to undertake

2. Identify which units will form the award

3. Identify which unit(s) you and your candidate will start work on

4. Devise and agree a learning contract/assessment plan for the unit(s)

5. Decide which teaching methods you will utilise to deliver the relevant underpinning knowledge

6. Decide which assessment methods you will utilise to determine overall competence

7. Teach and assess!

This process can be applied to any candidate undertaking any NVQ/SVQ, from an HCA undertaking level 2 in Care through to a registered nurse employed as a matron in a nursing home, undertaking the Residential Managers' award at level 4. Indeed, the principles of teaching and assessing are the same regardless of academic or vocational level or pathway.

An HCA may complete her NVQ with the main methods of assessment being direct observation and written questions, whereas a nursing student may be expected to produce some reflective accounts and critical analysis of scenarios, as well as being directly observed in practice. Likewise, a registered nurse undertaking study at master's level will be expected to complete some in-depth research.

# CONCLUSION

This chapter has provided you with information about how to evaluate and assess your students' learning in practice and should have enabled you to differentiate between the two. Practitioners who are teachers need to be fully committed to the process of evaluation, not only in relation to patient/client care, but also in relation to the students themselves, as it is the students who will, in the future, provide the high-quality care that we all seek to deliver.

# REFERENCES

Abbatt F, McMahon R. Teaching healthcare workers: a practical guide, 2nd edn. London: Macmillan, 1993

Andrew M. Using reflection to develop clinical expertise. British Journal of Nursing 1996; 5: 508–513

Benner P. From novice to expert. Menlo Park CA: Addison Wesley, 1984

Burnard P. Self evaluation methods in nurse education. Nurse Education Today 1988; 8: 229–233

Ellington H, Percival F, Race P. Handbook of educational technology, 3rd edn. London: Kogan Page, 1993

English National Board for Nursing, Midwifery and Health Visiting and Department of Health. Preparation of mentors and teachers: a new framework for guidance. London: English National Board, 2001

Kiger AM. Teaching for health, 2nd edn. New York: Churchill Livingstone, 1995

Nicklin PJ, Kenworthy N. Teaching and assessing in nursing practice: an experiential approach. Harcourt China, 2000

Nursing and Midwifery Council. The PREP handbook. London: NMC, 2002

QCA. Qualifications in England, Wales and Northern Ireland. QCA, 1997a

QCA. The awarding bodies' common accord. QCA, 1997b

Reece I, Walker S. Teaching and learning – a practical guide, 3rd edn. New College, Durham: Business Education Publishers, 1997

Rogers A. Teaching adults. Milton Keynes: Open University Press, 1994

Royal College of Nursing. Helping students get the best from their practice placements: a Royal College of Nursing toolkit. London: RCN, 2002

Storey L, Howard J, Gillies A. Competency in health care – a practical guide to competency frameworks. Oxford: Radcliffe Medical Press, 2002

UKCC (NMC). Standards for the preparation of teachers of nursing midwifery and health visiting. London: UKCC, 2000

Ward-Griffin C, Brown P. Evaluation of teaching – a review of the literature. Journal of Advanced Nursing 1992; 17: 1408–1414

# Index

Page numbers in **bold** refer to illustrations and tables